Chuck, Christa &
Jamie —

Thank you for your
Hospitality to the beautiful
Retreat! Our Chironwmy Rhythm
enjoyed our Time together Here. Let us know if we
plan to be back. Align our missions —
can Help
— Jvot

D0323469

THE ADJUSTMENT
ADVANTAGE

THE ADJUSTMENT ADVANTAGE

YOUR POTENTIAL FOR ACHIEVING A HIGHER QUALITY OF LIFE

TRENT SCHEIDECKER, DC

CHIR**O**WAY
CHIROPRACTIC

ChiroWay Chiropractic, LLC

The Adjustment Advantage:

A Small Spinal Alteration Co-Created By A Chiropractor To Achieve A Higher Quality Of Life.

CONTENTS

3

THE ART

DISCLAIMER

All content found in this publication, including: title, text, advice, or benefits were created for informational purposes only. The title is not stating any chiropractic practice, chiropractor, treatment or advice in this publication is more favorable or of superior position. Rather, when receiving Chiropractic Care one has an opportunity to gain a higher quality life or a favorable circumstance of lesser vertebral subluxation. The information in this book is not intended to diagnose, mitigate, or prescribe the use of any technique as a form of treatment for any physical conditions, symptoms, or diseases. Directly consult with a qualified health care professional for any medical, chiropractic questions or advice. All information and resources found in this publication are based on the opinions of the author and are meant to motivate and inform readers to make their own health decisions after consulting with their health care provider. In addition to the opportunity to gain a higher quality life or benefits of Chiropractic Care, one should also be aware of the existence of some risks. Risks associated with some Chiropractic Care may include soreness, musculoskeletal sprain/strain, and fracture. In addition, there have been reported cases of stroke associated with Chiropractic Care. Research and scientific evidence does not establish a cause and effect relationship between Chiropractic Care and the occurrence of stroke; rather studies indicate that people may be consulting chiropractors when they are in the early stages of a stroke. In essence, there is a stroke already in process. However, you are being informed of this reported risk. Trying to manipulate your own spine in an attempt to facilitate a Chiropractic Adjustment on yourself is not recommended. People may have the urge to "crack" their own spine in the hopes they'll receive momentary relief from the stiffness, tension, or pain that they are experiencing. If self-manipulation turns into a habit of temporary relief, problems can occur due to the potential negative effects this practice can create on the soft tissue ligaments, muscles and even facet joints. The author does not recommend or endorse any specific technique or form of treatment, Chiropractor, products, procedures, opinions, or other information that may be mentioned in this publication.

DEDICATION

This book is dedicated to my two children Tristan and Laila. The opportunity to serve you, The Adjustment Advantage for the past 8 years as a parent and Chiropractor has opened my eyes to how influential Regular Chiropractic Care is for the next generation of children to experience a higher quality of life. The day you were born, you were evaluated for vertebral subluxation and started to experience The Adjustment Advantage. This opportunity between the three of us has allowed me to clarify my professional recommendations for infants and children benefiting from Regular Chiropractic Care.

You two have confirmed my philosophy on how no two people are alike and no two Chiropractic Adjustments are alike. The differences in frequency, location, listings of vertebral subluxation, and response to the Chiropractic Adjustments you receive are enlightening and humbling. You two have been at the forefront of my passion to make Regular Chiropractic Easy Peasy Lemon Squeezy for the communities we serve at ChiroWay. Remember that as life goes on, so too does stress and that's when you need to reinvest even more proactive choices for your well-being. The potential is within you to live to your highest quality of life and I hope to see you both choose The Adjustment Advantage as one fundamental way to bring forth the innate power to adapt to the demands and stress that await you.

Parents, if you have not yet brought your children to have their spine analyzed for vertebral subluxation, consider this as an opportunity to learn more about Regular Chiropractic Care in the following pages.

INTRODUCTION

Have you ever considered how much potential you have within you? Have you ever thought how much potential is within your children? For example, the potential to heal a simple cut on your finger, or the potential within your child to heal their broken arm from falling at the park? Most of us take for granted the abilities that we all have residing within us. These abilities are powerful and untapped at most times due to the lack of recognition or interference to it.

The purpose of this book is to bring more awareness to the simple principle that we all have the potential to achieve a higher quality of life. This higher quality of life can be experienced by making small steps towards your desired potential. Your highest quality of life is like the potential energy of a ball waiting at the top of a hill. It's sitting there waiting to be expressed into another form of energy or higher quality of life. In order to convert your current condition to a higher quality, you need to make small alterations, or steps towards your desired potential. You need to take steps up the hill towards the top — the top of the hill is where the potential lies. These small alterations can be in many different forms.

These small alterations can come in forms of choosing to eat an apple a day or walking around the block every morning. Visiting your Chiropractor even when you feel good. Moving your body when you don't feel like it. Just one small alteration or step towards your desired potential that's waiting for you at the top of the hill. Since my background is within Chiropractic, I would like to propose a small alteration that can be made with a Chiropractor, The Adjustment Advantage.

The Adjustment Advantage is a small spinal alteration co-created by a Chiropractor to achieve a higher quality life.

The Adjustment Advantage is an investment into your well-being to reach toward a potential full of possibility that can express a higher quality of life. This book will address, in detail, how The Adjustment Advantage can enhance your inner potential towards a higher quality of life. However, due to the average person only reading one book a year, I'd like to give you a peek ahead by reinforcing the conviction I hold for the potential benefits of The Adjustment Advantage.

The Adjustment Advantage can be a safe and effective way to promote more well-being within the body. To get the most from The Adjustment Advantage, you must first grow in your understanding of the principles of Chiropractic so you can take the actions of incorporating it into your lifestyle. Your comprehension of the principles of Chiropractic can help produce greater results from The Adjustment Advantage by fully grasping how to use it to your advantage.

The philosophy behind The Adjustment Advantage is founded on the concept that your well-being is dependent upon a complete state of function coordinated by your neurological system.

All living organisms have three necessities of physiology: intelligence, matter and energy. The intelligence within the physiology is the guiding force of organization and coordination that allows our trillions of cells to work in a state of harmony throughout the body. The matter is our physical body of functioning systems that are built from cells, tissues and organs. The energy is the connection between the intelligence and matter that flows throughout the body, keeping you in a state of "being." Life energy travels to and from the brain through the nerves to all parts of the body. The energy source, coordinator and communicator to your well-being is how

The Adjustment Advantage can promote whole body benefits towards your desired potential or higher quality of life. Through the application of The Adjustment Advantage, interference in the life energy traveling through your neurological system can be removed. With the brain being the source of your life energy, it sends energy down the spinal cord and then out to your entire body through the nerves. This cycle then repeats back from the body through the nerves, up the spinal cord, and into the brain. This cyclical flow of energy from the brain to the body and the body back to the brain through your neurological system is how your trillions of cells work together physiologically.

When any of the 24 vertebrae subluxate out of proper position, interference in the transmission of life energy can occur between your brain and body. This is what chiropractors term "vertebral subluxation." The correction of vertebral subluxation is accomplished through The Adjustment Advantage, similar to turning the dimmer light switch up.

The Adjustment Advantage assists the vertebrae into normal alignment and function with gentle pressure in a specific line of drive. The Adjustment Advantage opens up the circuit between the brain and body by creating less interference in the neurological system, allowing normal function to occur throughout the entire body due to adequate nerve supply.

All parts of your body work in union with each other through the control and coordination of the neurological system. Your quality of life is a complexity of physical, mental and psychological states that combine to create an overall state of well-being. The three dimensions of your quality of life are interconnected through the neurological system and must be balanced to live optimally. If your neurological system is malfunctioning due to vertebral subluxation, your ability to reach your desired potential can be lessened.

The big idea behind The Adjustment Advantage is that there is a principle of physiological creation and restoration of new cells and tissues within us. This principle that runs the body, without any outside help, utilizes the neurological system for the coordination of trillions of cells working together. When the brain can communicate with the body without interference, the body can function in a state of ease similar to the ball sitting at the top of a hill, holding its potential energy within.

The Adjustment Advantage is a proactive choice to ensure optimal function within your spinal dynamics. Neglecting The Adjustment Advantage when needed, can diminish the potential results it has for you to experience. Similar to how the potential energy within the ball at the top of the hill is dependent upon how much conversion between potential and kinetic energy is taking place as it rolls down, the same is true for The Adjustment Advantage: the sooner you start, the more time you have to convert potential energy into kinetic energy.

1

THE PHILOSOPHY

"Why on earth should Chiropractic have a philosophy? Dentistry doesn't have a philosophy, Podiatry doesn't have a philosophy, Optometry doesn't have a philosophy, Medicine doesn't, Law doesn't, Architecture doesn't. Why in the world does Chiropractic need a Philosophy? The answer is; Chiropractic doesn't need a philosophy, Chiropractic is a philosophy."

- Reggie Gold, DC

| 1 |

MAJOR PREMISE

"The speculative method, by deduction, introspection
and hypothesis, erects elaborate structures of belief or
philosophy on slight foundations of fact. In this method
the processes are essentially subjective, deductive and
prior; the mind works from assumed cause to effect, from
subjective thought into the objective world. Great thinkers
in all ages have thus formulated complete schemes
covering whole departments of knowledge of the entire
universe, and have taken such pride in these brilliant
creations of their own intellects, and have regarded
them as so complete and perfect, that observation of
Nature was regarded as superfluous and unnecessary."

- B.J. Palmer

METHODOLOGY

Your life started with two microscopic cells uniting together for
creation of one cell, forming the foundation of all cells necessary in
your body. Only three weeks into your life, one of the very first organs

to develop was your neural tube which advanced into your neurological system: The brain and spinal cord.

You grew rapidly in the first four to eight weeks. At around six weeks, your neurological system underwent major development. Your spinal cord and brain sprouted out from the center of your body to all parts of your body forming tiny little buds at the end of each neurological shoot. These buds expanded and turned into your major organs, like your heart, lungs, stomach, arms, legs, and bones in your spine. Within your first eight weeks of life, you developed from a single cell life form to a one gram human body with all the major organs. You were about as big as four pinches of salt. After your first eight weeks of life you continued to transform into who you are now through rapid neurological synapses and migration throughout your body. This growth phase of your neurological system allowed your body to start moving and responding to stimuli. As you were growing through your first couple months of life, your body got stronger, and increased in length and weight.

This growth and development doesn't stop once you're born. You continued to develop after you were born. All of this growth and development took place rapidly and without the help of any outside forces, other than the intimate physiological connection to your mother for the first nine months. You grew from one cell to an estimated seventy trillion cells without any help! Just think about that for a minute. The amount of transformation that occurred within your body in the first couple years of life is astronomical when you consider the number of cells dividing and forming into their respective roles.

I hope this short description reminds you that you still have this transformative power within you to create new cells and tissues. All without the help of any outside forces. For example, think back to your last paper cut, bump, or bruise that left a mark to be seen. Now, put this book down and look at where that cut or bump took place. It's likely that it's not there anymore. What's the point?

The ability to transform from one cell into seventy trillion cells in the first 8 weeks of life is the point! The power of transformation and replication of new cells when you were growing inside your mother is the same power that turns your cut or bruise into new cells and tissues.

We all have this quality of life force within our body, and for many of us, we take it for granted or simply forget about the amazing physiological processes taking place within us everyday.

Not chiropractors though! Chiropractors are passionate about this quality of life force that's within us and we love to share the reminder with everyone we speak to that the body is self healing and self regulating. Self healing can be characterized by an innate recuperative power within the body.

The first chapter of this book is titled "MAJOR PREMISE" for a reason. Life is big. Life is astronomical. If you are willing to turn the microscope on it.

Understanding how vital your quality of life is, is the first principle you need to grasp before you can move onto the next chapter. They say you need to know where you are going in order to get there.

THIS IS TRUE FOR THE ADJUSTMENT ADVANTAGE. YOU NEED TO KNOW WHERE THE DESTINATION IS, BEFORE YOU CAN BEGIN MAKING ADJUSTMENTS TOWARDS IT.

It's about the method. The methodology to gaining a higher quality life needs to be constructively criticized. Life, or the state of being alive, is the destination. But, being alive is fluctuating and ever changing.

For instance, cells are constantly turning over, dying, and regenerating in your body due to wear and tear. This process is most common in the blood and digestive tract, due to the immune system being heavily concentrated within the blood. Some cells in your body have a lifespan as short as a day. They can be considered the first line of defense. The current estimates for cell turnover within an average person's body is between 50-70 billion cells per day! The current guess on the amount of total cells in your body is currently 70 trillion. So, 50-70 billion cells out of your 70 trillion cells are turning over, dying, and regenerating every single day!

This amount of change means that our destination for co-creating a higher quality of life is a moving target. You can't hit the bullseye as easily when the target keeps disappearing and reappearing in a new location. If the destination is in constant motion, then our focus needs to change from the results to the process.

The process is the journey. The journey is the transformation. Being alive is exactly that: it's a journey of being. Being is transformative, and in order to co-create a higher quality of life, we need to look further into the principles that make up being alive so we can have a complete grasp of what choices to make that will benefit our body to the fullest degree.

Quality of life can be defined as the standard of health, comfort and happiness experienced by an individual. Your quality of life and how you experience it is greatly impacted by the standard of your overall well-being.

How do you measure life in the context of your health or well-being? How do you measure the current state of being alive within your body?

What's the current methodology to know for certain how much life we have within us? Measuring how much life or your quality of life that is within the body is not easy to do. Measuring if there is a lack of life within the body is easier to do.

Current processes for tracking and monitoring well-being typically fall under the observation of statistical averages and seeing where you are in the bell curve compared to the rest of the population being measured. For children, growth rate is a process that is used to monitor the child's growth and development compared to other children. Growth rate calculations determine if the child falls within the average growth rate compared to other children. Growth rate measures the height, weight and head circumference, and compares that to the average growth rate of other children. Based on where your child falls in the statistics of the bell curve, this information is used as a parameter or assessment of malnutrition or illness that might be interfering with growth.

What if the child's weight is in the ninety-ninth percentage on the growth rate chart compared to other children? Does that mean the child is ninety-nine percent full of life? Or, does it mean the child is one percent less likely to have malnutrition or illness present? These are two different questions if you re-read them. The objective of growth monitoring consists of routine measurement to detect abnormal growth. Detecting abnormal growth is the objective. This objective is different from saying the growth rate is a measurement to detect normal growth. The methodology to monitor abnormal vs. normal are two different methods.

Monitoring vital signs is another process for measuring and detecting if anything is abnormal within the body. Vital signs such as body temperature, heart rate, respiratory rate and blood pressure assess the life sustaining functions of the body. They help determine current diseases or if future adverse outcomes are possible. Measuring to detect abnormality in the body can be a life saving procedure. Unfortunately, my grandfather did not benefit from this form of measuring abnormality within the body and passed away at the age of 52.

When he suffered his first heart attack, it was too late to do anything further to keep him alive. His first major symptom was his last symptom. Did he have other indicators that could have projected the seriousness of the state of condition for his heart and overall health? If we could go back to that time in his life and take his vitals, I would take an educated guess that there would have been indicators that would have led us to believe his heart was under stress. There might have been abnormal warning signs within his vitals.

These indicators are great when you're pressing the outer limits of the methodology of monitoring abnormal. They are not statistically significant when monitoring how normal the physiology is functioning. The two methods are different. The objective is to detect abnormality within the body, to detect if something has deviated from the normal statistic compared to the rest being measured. Metrics that fall outside the realm of average compared to those being measured will quantify if there is something wrong with your body. What measurement can constitute how much quality of life or well-being there is within your human framework? In order to better answer that question, we have to understand the systematic and logical approach of viewing how our body functions.

REASONING

While searching for answers to questions like how do we quantify quality of life or being alive, you have to start the process by creating theories. Theories in the realm of what causes what and why.

Many professional fields are formed around a revolutionary theory that proves to change the current mindset to a new way of thinking, a paradigm shift. This process is usually a reorganization of current knowledge into a new order that answers a question that was unanswered before. This reorder of information requires your mindset to be open to receiving this information in order for you to accept it.

One of the most impactful theories that not only revolutionized the way we do things on a day to day basis, but also the use of the word revolution itself, was the theory of heliocentrism. This theory was developed by an ancient Greek astronomer Nicolaus Copernicus. Nicolaus Copernicus developed and convinced us of the theory that the earth revolves around the center of the solar system: the sun. Nicolaus Copernicus' theory was revolutionary as it was exactly the opposite of what the Roman Catholic Church aligned with: the sun revolving around the earth. Before his theory was proven as truth, the accepted knowledge was that the sun revolved around the earth.

This sounds ridiculous, but the reorganization of the knowledge at that time took massive effort and was resisted by many because of what was accepted as truth. He stood alone in defense of it against the current mindset at that time and his theory proved to be true.

Theories are tested and evaluated, whether they are true or not, within a branch of knowledge or philosophy. Branches of knowledge or philosophy is a classification of wisdom by those who study these theories within the context of that branch. For example, metaphysics is a branch of knowledge that studies theories within the context of nature of existence and reality. Epistemology is the branch of knowledge that deals with nature and knowledge. Ethics is a branch of knowledge that studies what's right or wrong. Logic is the branch of knowledge that studies theories of correct reasoning. These branches of knowledge are a collection of information for the search for truth or facts. Branches of knowledge are valuable within professional industries as they become a resource for the practical application of the theory. Theories can turn into applications whether they are true or false. When the application of a false theory is commonplace, it takes time and further clarification and reorganization of the information to develop a new and hopefully correct theory.

The original theory of being pronounced dead was based on whether a person was still breathing. In 1798, German priest P.G. Pessler proposed that all coffins have a cord running through a hole that would be connected to the church bells. The person who was pronounced dead, because they were no longer breathing, would be buried with the cord in hand and if they came back to life they could ring the church bells. This proposal sparked the idea of creating coffins that had signaling systems or "safety coffins." Safety coffins were a physical sign that the accepted theory of being dead was not true. It wasn't uncommon for people to be buried alive not all that long ago because of the false theory that you were dead when you stopped breathing. This theory has now been replaced with proven concepts in medicine that the human body is no longer alive when brain activity ceases.

The current explanation of death is based on the organ that sustains life within the body: the neurological system. The neurological system is the first "organ" to develop in your body and it's the coordinating organ that connects all your cells, tissues and organs together so there is a harmonious action of function that can occur.

As much knowledge as we've attained on how the human body functions, we still don't have all the answers for how the body works. It's been stated by Thomas Edison "We don't know a millionth of one percent about anything." I believe that quote still holds validity today as it did then in relation to human physiology. We don't know everything about the human body!

Our lack of understanding means we look at all the facts we've found and come up with the wrong conclusions. Our limited perspective looks at A and B and thinks A caused B, when maybe we're not looking at the proper relationship with cause and effect.

A vivid illustration of coming to the wrong conclusions includes the practice of bloodletting. The oldest theories of good health revolved around the idea that blood had to be in perfect balance or state. If sickness was evident, the practice of draining blood from your body would get rid of the bad blood and sickness with it. Bloodletting became the standard approach to treating ill health and was even performed on America's first president, George Washington. Bloodletting was more harmful than beneficial in the cases that were documented throughout its longevity. This evidence has proved the theory of getting rid of sickness through the blood to be false.

Our society makes decisions based on knowledge, and in some circumstances the wrong knowledge. Knowledge isn't enough to move you towards a higher quality of life. The understanding of the knowledge is what's necessary. There is so much information in this world and knowing the information is good, but good isn't good enough. Understanding the information is the difference between burying a person who isn't breathing but still alive and burying a person who isn't breathing and is dead in a coffin.

Looking back on all the knowledge we thought we understood but didn't, reveals the necessity for complete comprehension of accurate knowledge. Living a life of incomplete understanding is an injustice to your true potential. You may think all is well, but then realize you had incomplete understanding when signs and symptoms finally appear due to the compounding effects of time and stress.

Understanding accurate knowledge equals greater performance. Greater performance in making decisions will move you towards the right outcomes. Making the right decisions because you understand the principle of that knowledge is a form of educated adaptation. You're choosing which direction to move to not only for your survival, but for the ability to thrive. Understanding knowledge allows you to adapt to the demands and stressors of your life that try to break you down.

Greater performance and adapting to life's demands can add longevity to your life. By making the right decisions for your well-being with the information you hold, you are able to take advantage of the positive effects that come through health care, work environment, relationships with others, and all factors that contribute to your well-being.

UNDERSTANDING ACCURATE KNOWLEDGE AND MAKING THE RIGHT DECISION WHEN FACED WITH A CHOICE IS BASED ON TWO FUNDAMENTALS: INDUCTIVE REASONING AND DEDUCTIVE REASONING.

Inductive and deductive reasoning are opposite forms of logical reasoning when trying to understand knowledge.

Inductive reasoning is used when the facts are not available - you are acting on what you assume the facts to be. Inductive reasoning is a thought process for creating conclusions based on a prediction from observing something that is true. It's a way of logically forecasting from part to whole or small to large. For example: all living things require water to exist, therefore in order to find new life it will be dependent upon water to exist. Inductive reasoning is a great way to create hypotheses and theories in the scientific model when all variables are known and consistent. The limitation to using this logical evidence based practice in human physiology is the body has many possible internal and external factors that cannot possibly be accounted for every time. When all factors are not included, you have false positives or false negatives. People are also slightly different from each other and the law of individuality should be recognized when applying a hypothesis or theory to the human body.

Just the mere fact of recognizing that the statement may be true, but it may not, is a step in the direction of realizing you need more than one way of thinking to complete the whole picture. If inductive reasoning has shortcomings and is the opposite of deductive reasoning, then utilizing deductive logic along with the inductive method would help you understand the information better. Alternating between inductive and deductive reasoning will form more complete conclusions.

DEDUCTION

Deductive reasoning is used when you use the facts to create your knowledge. While you try to make informed decisions, or understand everything someone is sharing with you, or research you find, utilizing deductive reasoning with your understanding is a thinking process that will build your actions on foundations of principles and facts. Deductive reasoning starts with a major principle or premise that is without any doubt true, and then from there you deduce other principles that must be true because the major premise is true. An example of the power of deductive reasoning is as follows; major premise: my dog always barks when she hears someone at the door. Deduced conclusion: My dog is not barking right now so no one is at the door. Deductive reasoning was used in Chiropractic by stating a major premise that cannot be denied and logically concluding statements that must also be true by reasoning from the major premise. This was useful early on in our development of our profession while we were building certainty, but is just as powerful now as it was over one-hundred years ago. Knowledge is power, but it has limits when it relates to the human body. Accepting the fact we don't have all the answers as to how the body functions to make up a complete state of quality of life, can move us in the direction of seeking greater understanding of the information that we do have.

The benefit of searching for understanding of how our body functions lies in Aristotle's statement that "The whole is more than the sum of its parts." The whole body is greater than the sum of its parts. What this means is the individual parts of your body are connected together to form your body as a complete entity, they are worth more than if the parts were alone. The parts of your body require each other to function; they are connected together by an unquantifiable recuperative force that coordinates the body parts to keep the parts working in harmony. This principle of coordination within us is unquantifiable. This coordinating recuperative power within our body is unquantifiable because it can't be measured as a quantity.

If we leave unquantifiable measurements out of the equation, it's now an incomplete equation that will produce facts out of context. Taking facts out of context makes it an informal fallacy. Since we cannot quantify how the sum of the body functions, because of the fact that there are unquantifiable features to being alive, and that the whole is greater than the sum of its parts. Using deductive reasoning to understand how your body's quality of life can be quantified is your next best step in moving towards a higher quality of life.

We do know with certainty that in order to function, our body is structured with the necessity of the heart, kidneys, liver, lungs and brain to be operating properly. For this reason, these organs are termed "vital" or "essential." The heart is in charge of circulating blood throughout the body to supply cells, tissues and organs with oxygen and energy. Every cell in our body requires oxygen, removal of carbon dioxide and a constant supply of energy. The heart's responsibility of beating millions of times through its lifetime is structured as a musculature pump in order to perform its vital function. The kidneys have the responsibility to excrete waste and fluids so we don't over hydrate or fill up with toxins. The kidneys are our filtration system: they excrete the unnecessary and keep what's essential. The structure of the kidneys filtration system matches the primary responsibility of keeping our blood pressure in chemical balance. The liver's multiple functions revolve around detoxification and production of digestive enzymes. It's the second largest organ in the body, skin being the first. The structure of the liver is to receive blood through its thousands of lobules that consist of veins, arteries and sinusoids to detoxify the blood and production of bile for digestion. The lungs allow us to take oxygen from the air and incorporate it into our blood while removing carbon dioxide from the blood preventing toxic levels. The anatomy and structure of the lungs is a spongy air filled organ with the capabilities to exchange molecules of oxygen between air and blood. The brain is the entire body's control center, keeping our trillions of cells working as one unit. It's the coordinating organ to the rest of the body's vital organs through constant communication of information through the neurological system. The reception and employment of neurological impulses allows us to adapt to our daily functions, like breathing, heart rate and digestion, and keep the body working together.. The structure of the brain and neurological system is designed for storing and transmitting information.

The astonishing functions of the human body through its vital organs produce extraordinary facts. There are estimates that there are over one-hundred trillion cells within our body! Just so you can actually comprehend how large one-hundred trillion cells are, let's use time as an analogy. A trillion seconds would equal thirty-two thousand years. If each cell in your body equaled a second in time, you have thirty two thousand years of cells within you!

The capability of over one-hundred trillion cells functioning together, and separately for their specific physiological purpose is hard to fathom. It's so mind staggering, that we don't know all the facts about the human body. Not having all the facts, but knowing some facts, can still be crafted together to create a level of understanding. Utilizing deductive reasoning to conclude more facts from the major premise can be an effective approach to grasping how the body functions in a complete state of optimal well-being.

We know for a fact that all physical matter in the universe, including our physical body is composed of atoms. Atoms are units of energy formed from protons, electrons and neutrons. The number of electrons that differ from one atom to the next is what makes matter different from one form to the next. The electrons are the primary carrier of energy and are interchangeable with matter itself; $E=mc^2$. We can conclude from all of the facts that all matter has atoms and in order for matter to exist, there needs to be an organization to the electrons around the atom. This fact that organization exists within atoms and matter itself can indicate another principle for you to use in understanding how to co-create a higher quality of life within the body.

> ORGANIZATION INDICATES THAT INTELLIGENCE IS PRESENT; WE KNOW FOR FACT THAT INTELLIGENCE EXISTS DUE TO THE PRESENCE OF ORGANIZATION. INTELLIGENCE IS A PROPERTY OF ORGANIZATION. THE TWO REQUIRE EACH OTHER TO EXIST.

From the conclusion that atoms make up the universe and there is organization to each atom, we can create a major premise that is undeniable and can be used as a reference for deducing other facts. R.W. Stephenson in 1927 wrote a book titled, "*The Chiropractic Textbook*" and within the text he copyrighted the major premise to the practice of Chiropractic: "A Universal Intelligence is in all matter and continually gives to it all its properties and actions, thus maintaining it in existence."

Recognizing that there is organization throughout the universe, including our human body, is the starting point of understanding how The Adjustment Advantage can enhance your quality of life.

This organization leads us to deduce that there is a Universal Intelligence that is in all matter and continually gives to it all its properties and actions, thus maintaining it in existence. Albert Einstein made the observation, "the more we understand nature, the more we can comprehend how these universal principles apply to us."

The definition of intelligence centers around the ability to acquire and or apply knowledge or information. We use intelligence to describe the universe due to the observation that atoms and molecules that exist throughout the universe are bundles of energy expressing information. Not information in the sense of facts, but rather arrangements or sequences that show organization. The universe is intelligently organized. There is some randomness, but the harmony that exists is the foundation to how everything works together.

To demonstrate this Universal Intelligence, let's observe plants and the process of the seed growing into maturity. Roots always shoot down into the soil, not up into the air where they wouldn't flourish. Leaves don't hide in the shade, but always reach towards the light for the aid of more growth. Leaves drop from trees during the cold dry months that don't produce enough water to sustain the vegetation. Each growing branch on a tree turns away from the other in search of more room for growth rather than fighting the next branch which is ultimately connected to the same tree. This example of nature and organization is a way of seeing that there isn't random action, but rather intelligence expressing itself universally.

| 2 |

INNATE INTELLIGENCE

"The Chiropractor assumes an entirely broader
viewpoint. There is no question but that the laws of
Chemistry and Physics are involved in the functioning of the
human body. But, these laws of Chemistry and Physics are
in turn governed and controlled by a higher power, an
immaterial force which we have called
Innate (inborn) Intelligence."

- D.D. Palmer

ORDER

How often have you tried to discuss a topic with someone who just wouldn't budge on their viewpoint? You try reasoning with them to see it from your perspective, but with no success. Often people's perspectives on topics are held together by a major premise that they stand firmly behind.

Say you're having a conversation with a family member about how important it is to visit a chiropractor on a regular basis, due to all the benefits you've seen from it in your personal life. You could tell them until you're blue in the face about how significant of a difference you've experienced in your quality of life, but they just don't budge in their actions.

Why is this? Is it because they don't "believe you?" Or is it because their major premise about well-being lies on a different proposition than yours?

Maybe their major premise about their body is to seek help from a health care provider only when the body can't perform its daily functions. In other words, when it's completely broken down, only then do they look for help to fix it. If the way you choose to invest into your well-being is founded on a different major premise than those you are trying to convert to your way, chances are you will have little success converting. You won't be able to push them towards a proactive choice for their quality of life if they only operate on a reactive major premise.

Understanding that Universal Intelligence is in all matter and continually gives all its properties and actions, thus maintaining it in existence, is important as we move on to the next philosophical principle that supports The Adjustment Advantage. If there is intelligence within every aspect of the universe, then that must mean our body has intelligence within it. We can deduce this truth about this principle by deriving it from the whole: the major premise.

The body is full of intelligence, both Educated and Innate Intelligence. The Educated Intelligence is that which we gain through life; the Innate Intelligence is that which we are born with. The common Chiropractic illustration of Innate Intelligence is that for nine months, an infant inside a mother requires very little help to grow into a living breathing baby from anything other than the mother's supply of nutrients and warmth. The day the baby is born, we believe that the baby needs more help from the educated man who has learned through the years of studying babies, rather than looking to the wisdom that resides within the baby. The same wisdom that turned two cells into one and then into trillions in just a couple months time. Yes, the innate intelligence within every living breathing body is full of wisdom that keeps the body alive and functioning as one harmonious organism. The point of the illustration and for you to become aware of the inner wisdom within your body that is striving for adaptable conditions. Albert Einstein concluded his professional career with a question that is case in point to the inner wisdom that is striving for adaptation. Albert Einstein asked this enlightening question in search of clarifying his major premise during research: "The most important question you can ever ask is if the Universe is a friendly place?"

Ask yourself right now, is this Universe friendly or hostile? What comes to mind? Both? Can there be both? Does it have to be one or the other? From a physicist viewpoint, which is built on laws or principles that are true or false, it can only be one or the other. The universe is either a friendly universe or a hostile universe. In the world of principles, equations are used to support the question being asked. For instance, $E=mc^2$ is the equation that supports the question of whether or not energy can be created or destroyed. When searching for the answer to where energy comes from, a major premise was clarified: it's neither created nor destroyed. It can only be transferred or interchanged. The definition of Universe is, "all existing matter and space considered as a whole." Does matter and the space that the matter lives in provide a perfect environment for more of what's in it? Does the Universe support life? These are big questions, but the easiest way to answer them would be to answer them in context of true or false. Is the Universe friendly? True or false?

We can answer that big question by looking at the scenario if the Universe was not friendly. Assuming the Universe is not friendly, all the matter and space that occupies this world would then be hostile. The food you ate would be hostile. The air you breathed would be hostile. The body you live in would be hostile. Everything would be antagonistic towards the support of order, harmony and organization. Are you painting a picture in your head right now that this isn't the answer to the question "is the Universe friendly or hostile?" This Universe is friendly!

If the matter which includes your cells and tissues and the food you eat, was not friendly or perfect, and did not support life in existence, you wouldn't be here. The Universe would not be supporting you right as you read these lines. That answer comes from an all or none, or true or false perspective: it's either friendly or hostile. If it's hostile, it would break down all your healthy cells and tissues and create nothing. There would be no further growth or sustainability. The apple you ate today would not be digested, assimilated and turned into healthy living cells and tissues if the Universe was hostile or unfriendly.

The question on whether or not this Universe is friendly or hostile does not mean that all matter and the space that matter occupies is constantly performing as it strives for support and order. Yes, there are hostile conditions within this Universe. Yes, there are malfunctioning parts within the human body. Yes, we only live, on average, 80 years until the body breaks down and cannot carry on its functions. There is hostility within this Universe, but just because something is unfavorable, does not indicate that all matter is striving for hostility. The visible areas in this Universe where matter is not working perfectly is a sign that something is interfering with the perfection towards friendly conditions. The Universe is friendly, that means it is constantly striving for organization or a state of condition of being free, or as free as possible from defects. Defects and imperfection do exist, but the Universe is not searching for imperfection and disharmony. That would be a self-destructive universe. In order to reach a higher quality of life or your desired potential for more well-being, the viewpoint of whether or not your body is striving for inner perfection and is healing towards health and wholeness is vital to your success. You will not attain the perfect condition of strength, vitality and overall well-being if you philosophically believe that the Universe is hostile.

True, there is danger within the world. There are chemicals that can hurt the body and there is daily stress that will break down your mind. Along with these negative forces and stressors to our body there resides limitations to the amount of resistance to the forces we can withstand. The more force or stressors, the more likely our positive nature of health and healing cannot adapt. Those are all facts, but what is also true in this viewpoint of well-being and health is there is an inner perfection trying to adapt to those external invasive forces that are breaking down cells and tissues. This inner perfection strives for a friendly state of health and structure. It strives for more cells and tissues that work together. There is an Innate Intelligence within your body that constantly strives to make the body to be as good as it can possibly be.

For example, every contraction and relaxation of your diaphragm is supported with a mental impulse from the Phrenic Nerve to and from your brain.

"Phrenic" means relating to the diaphragm. The Phrenic Nerve communicates to your diaphragm via impulses to help coordinate breathing. When you breathe in, your diaphragm "contraction" moves downward, making your chest expand and draw in more oxygen for your lungs. When you breathe out, your diaphragm "relaxes," allowing your chest to shrink back to a small size. Your Phrenic Nerve exits out of your neck around the C3-C5 region and travels down towards your lungs and heart to supply vital mental impulses through the nerve to your diaphragm. An average person can have their diaphragm flex and relax about 16 times per minute, which means you take in about 23,000 breaths a day and, on average, over 8 million times per year!

What's the value of knowing about your Phrenic Nerve, diaphragm contraction and relaxation? The value lies in understanding that in order to properly breathe your average 16 breaths per minute, there is an Innate Intelligence guiding your well-being through neurological impulses between your brain and diaphragm.

There is more to these neurological impulses than just an impulse that says "breathe" or "contract diaphragm." There is intelligence within the impulse that causes a force to be expressed to the tissue of the diaphragm that coordinates proper contraction and relaxation for the right amount at the right time. The Innate Intelligence of the body not only protects the body from invasive forces, but it also produces coordination and harmony around the clock.

Production is defined as the action of making or manufacturing from components or raw materials.

Our body takes in raw materials from the food we eat, or even the air we breathe in, and manufactures health for our overall well-being.

The ability to produce something from nothing (raw material) is how well-being is achieved. You don't find more health and well-being in a bottle or pill. You find it from the inside-out. Yes, the bottle or pill may aid and assist your production and even be the key factor in the process, but the production of more well-being in principle occurs within you. You are a well-being producing organism through the inner recuperative power of the body to intelligently recreate more living breathing tissue!

> INNATE IS A WORD THAT MEANS "BEING BORN WITH IT." IN CHIROPRACTIC, IT DIFFERENTIATES THE LIVING FROM THE NONLIVING.

In our human body, there is an Innate Intelligence that is actively keeping us in a state of organization. The simplest way to comprehend Innate Intelligence is by referring to it as a principle or law similar to the law of gravity.

Newton's law of gravity is defined as, "any particle in the universe attracts every other particle in the universe with a force which is directly proportional to the product of their masses and inversely proportional to the square of distance between their centers." This definition is a law or principle that was created within the branch of knowledge known as physics. The law of gravity is a principle that you cannot physically see, touch, or taste. It's an observation that works whether you believe it or not.

Innate intelligence is similar to the law of gravity in the respect that you can't see, touch, or taste it. It's not physical, it's a principle of truth. It is an observation that works within your body whether you believe it or not. Innate intelligence is not a theological term. Theology is the study of Christian teaching. Innate intelligence is a principle that was logically deduced, "deductive reasoning," from the major premise of Chiropractic over one-hundred years ago. In essence, it's a philosophical term to describe the active organization in a human body starting at the atomic level and working its way up through cellular, tissue, organ and even system organization. Your body is intelligently organized for the greater good of thriving in a complete state of harmony.

ORGANIZATION

Another way to make sense of Innate Intelligence is by taking a greater look at organization within our body. Biology recognizes that there are levels of organization, with the atom being the most basic essence of organization. As you bring together more matter (atoms), the level of complexity increases from the simplest unit of the atom to more complex degrees of organization. This begins with the simplest form of molecules, moving up in complexity to organelles, cells, and tissues which create organs, organ systems and finally, your entire body.

All of these levels of organization are held together by the principle of what Chiropractic refers to as Innate Intelligence. Where there is organization there is intelligence, the two are inseparable. Your body's Innate intelligence can be visualized when you look at the magnificent capabilities your vital organs play to keep you in a state of harmony. Your brain is coordinating the entire body's trillions of cells, while your heart is supplying oxygen and energy through the bloodstream. At the same time, your kidneys are excreting waste and fluids, your liver is detoxifying and producing digestive enzymes and your lungs allow you to take in oxygen and remove carbon dioxide from the bloodstream.

Your body functions with organization, which means you have an internal wisdom, or Innate Intelligence, that is expressing this organization. The unique aspect of living organisms is the ability to actively stay organized. When we compare the organization of a rock to a human body, both have atomic organization, but the rock lacks the ability to actively organize like the human body. If you break the rock in half, it remains broken and there is no active organization that brings it back together. If you break a bone in the human body, there is active organization towards healing. This active organization is a subset of Universal Intelligence and in Chiropractic we call it "Innate Intelligence."

Innate intelligence is intangible just like Universal Intelligence, so we need to look at the signs of Innate Intelligence to better comprehend this Chiropractic principle. R.W. Stephenson, DC documented five signs of life in 1948 in his book, "*The Chiropractic Textbook.*"

The five signs of Innate Intelligence within the body are: assimilation, excretion, adaptability, growth and reproduction. These five signs reinforce the rationalization that there is an intelligence or an inborn wisdom in the human body keeping your quality of life working in harmony.

LOOKING AT THE ACTIVE ORGANIZATION IN EACH SIGN OF LIFE CAN INCREASE YOUR AWARENESS OF THE SIMPLE CONCEPT THAT THE HUMAN BODY IS STRIVING TOWARDS WHOLENESS AND WELL-BEING.

The first sign of Innate Intelligence in your body is the power to selectively assimilate food. This process of selecting the nutrients that are needed at a specific moment in time is not random. The constant ability of gauging the chemical content of food requires intelligence within the body. If there was no intelligent assimilation taking place in your body, the pharmaceutical industry would be disproved. Pharmacy is based on predicting what chemical is needed or not needed in your body when it is introduced, and allowing your body's Innate Intelligence to assimilate that chemical for a desired purpose. Assimilation requires a constant active organization in order to judge what chemical or nutrient is needed at that specific time.

The second sign of Innate Intelligence in your body is the power to selectively excrete waste and toxins that are not necessary. When food goes into the body, active organization and monitoring of the toxins and waste levels are taking place so the body doesn't fill up with unnecessary chemicals that can hurt normal physiology. For example, what happens when you eat spoiled food? Your body likely goes into excretion mode to get rid of the toxins that were in the spoiled food.

The third sign of Innate Intelligence in your body is the power of adaptability. Adaptation in biology is the ability to change or respond to forces for overall survival in the environment. The key point to adaptation is response. The body can be placed in a new environment, discern the temperature and perspire to cool the body or shiver to warm it back up. Biologists and anthropologists have been studying adaptation in the human body as it relates to its environment and have concluded that there is active organization taking place for the overall well-being of the human body through adaptation.

The fourth sign of Innate Intelligence in your body is the power of growth. Growth requires active organization in order for size and direction to be controlled. If there is a lack of control in growth, this can become deadly. Growth has to be at the precise amount and time. Growth requires intelligence for the body's overall well-being, otherwise it can be a deadly force if left unchecked.

The fifth and final sign of Innate Intelligence in your body is the power of reproduction. Reproduction of the entire human body from one cell to trillions that make up one living breathing human body. This sign of life demonstrates that in order to be alive, you must have a plan to preserve life from oblivion or extinction. This sign is similar to growth, but more specifically in regards to the entire human race. The body can be in growth mode and reproduction mode at the same time, hence both are unique signs of Innate Intelligence.

AWARENESS

All of these signs that guide the body in an active state of organization are ways for us to consider how the body functions in a normal state. We need to understand how the body naturally works in order to know how it gets back to normal when deviation or injury takes place. If you're a typical adult, then you likely spend the day running from one task to the next.

Sometimes life moves so fast we lose track of our body and how it's responding and adapting to day to day demands and stressors. When this happens and life is moving faster than our awareness can keep up with, chances are that the choices you're making at that time may not be in your body's best interest. Making decisions while unaware of the positive or negative consequences is similar to making choices while having no knowledge of the situation or facts.

How often do we spend our days staying too busy to slow down and smell the roses? How about slowing down and becoming aware of the innate needs of your body? The challenge is to stay aware of your body during the busy times so you can make the intelligent choices for your well-being.

The faster we move, the more we demand of ourselves, the more we demand of ourselves requires us to become more aware. Aware of what it is that our body needs right now. The challenge of being aware of your body during demanding days is real. The busier you are, the tougher it is to make intelligent choices that can enhance your over-all well-being. Becoming more aware of your body is a goal everyone should challenge themselves to, and is a potential benefit from The Adjustment Advantage.

The body's Innate Intelligence allows its 70 trillion cells to function together as one operating body. Chiropractors have been discussing and debating Innate Intelligence for over one hundred years. Let's discuss the question "How can we benefit from becoming more aware of the body's Innate Intelligence?"

All living body's have an intelligence built within to guide the molecules and atoms into coordinated action. The organization bespeaks intelligence and strives towards overall function for the greater good of the body. In essence, Innate Intelligence is a principle. A principle or law like the law of gravity. It's there and it's working even though we can't see it. The Innate Intelligence of the body is where wisdom resides for the number of heart beats needed, which nutrients to digest and which to eliminate, and inner immunity to fight off the harmful infections and stress that our inner world fights every day through white blood cells and the rest of the immune cells. The Innate Intelligence of the body has this inner wisdom that knows more than our Educated Intelligence. Similar to the powerful statement Carl Jung made, "Who looks outside, dreams; who looks inside, awakes."

Looking inward can often bring a higher state of awareness to the challenges or questions you have. Imagine yourself waking up and in a state of hunger. You just slept for eight hours and you need to replenish your body with the appropriate nutrition to get the day started.

If you ask yourself what you're hungry for and all you can think about is having a banana and an orange, perhaps that may be a sign that you need Potassium and Vitamin C. Self awareness of your current needs can be done on more levels than just nutrition. You could do this same exercise for sleep, exercise, and other health promoting activities that your body requires.

The next time you have to decide, what should I do? Try looking inward and you may become aware of the needs of your well-being. In the search for your highest quality of life, gaining a wealth of knowledge on well-being, physiology and health, by looking inward can allow you to make more accurate predictions on what the future may hold.

President Abraham Lincoln is credited for saying "The best way to predict the future is to create it." Creating the future with your quality of life is reflected by the decisions you make, and the decisions you make are based on the knowledge you hold.

What is knowledge? Plato defined knowledge as "justified true belief." Another definition of knowledge is "facts, information, and skill acquired by a person through experience or education."

A SECRET TO SUCCESS WITH THE ADJUSTMENT ADVANTAGE IS UNDERSTANDING THAT SEEING IS BELIEVING. THE ACT OR EXPERIENCE OF DOING IT CREATES KNOWLEDGE.

If you see how it works for yourself, you will believe it to be true. I've been actively pursuing a higher quality of life for years. Every time I choose to invest into my well-being, I find myself experiencing a new level of strength and vitality that could not be explained through a prediction — the prediction becomes the act of experiencing it from the inside-out. Chiropractors have a saying, above-down-inside-out. Experiencing optimal well-being can come from above-down-inside-out.

A quote by Lao Tzu states, "Those who have knowledge, don't predict. Those who predict, don't have knowledge." Perhaps Lao Tzu is saying that you can't just talk or think about what it will be like, you have to experience it to know it.

A body working more efficiently allows your Educated Intelligence to focus on the day and on your body. This concept is similar to a wifi connection that is free of interference — your computer will allow you to efficiently download and play a Netflix video to your device. If the wifi is being interfered with, due to other devices streaming videos, you may lose proper playback to the video.

Greater adaptability through a higher functional neurological system can enhance your ability to pay attention to where you are and what's around you. How fast is life going? What is your body adapting to? Become aware of the ground you stand on, the air you're breathing in and the people who surround you. The foundation to reaching your highest quality of life resides in the knowledge that the body has the powerful innate ability to heal itself. Because the neurological system coordinates every cell and organ in your body, the structure of the spine being properly aligned influences a higher level of well-being. Give yourself an opportunity to predict the best case scenario for your future by creating it through positive decisions, and by looking for those innate needs through your innate awareness to lead you in the direction of your desired potential.

The Chiropractic major premise cannot be denied due to its conclusion from principles that are true. The purpose of having a major premise and principles in the Chiropractic profession is to create fundamental truths, or a position that serves as the backbone or foundation for a system of belief and reasoning. These Chiropractic principles are the foundation for the philosophy, science and art of Chiropractic. These principles are what the following chapters are built on, for you to learn how The Adjustment Advantage can influence a higher quality of life.

The study of these universal principles starts and stops there in the field of Chiropractic. We do not try to comprehend what this Universal Intelligence is, such as applying theoretical terms to it as God or the Supreme Being. Chiropractic is not a religion, it's a professional service centered around principles that support the services being offered.

There is no way to display Innate Intelligence due to being a principle or immaterial, it's similar to the law of gravity. You can deny gravity all you want, but if you jump off a bridge and say gravity doesn't exist, gravity doesn't stop existing. You'll still be brought down regardless of your belief in it. Logical reasoning or rationalization is how we comprehend this premise that there is organization throughout the universe. The principle of Innate Intelligence is great to discuss and comprehend from a physiological and philosophical viewpoint, but how do you apply it? The next step is acknowledging how the Innate Intelligence within the body raises your quality of life from the inside-out. Here are 3 Recommendations to Increase your Innate Awareness of Your Innate Needs:

1. Be Aware of Your Breathing. When life is pulling you out of rhythm, and chaos is in control, slow down the distracting thoughts and stress by being aware of your breathing. Breathing has an innate rhythmic process that can put you back in touch with how your body is adapting or compensating to the demands of the day.

2. Be Aware of Your Senses. Your body has five senses: sight, hearing, smell, taste and touch. Being aware of natural beauty around you like sunsets, the sounds of the songs you like to listen to, the smell of coffee or diffused essential oils, the taste of the food you're consuming throughout the day and the everyday textures of what you're touching will keep your awareness more alive!

3. Experience The Adjustment Advantage. One way, but not the only way, of investing into well-being and becoming more aware

of the innate needs is regular Chiropractic Adjustments. Chiropractic Adjustments focused on the facilitation of removing vertebral subluxation can influence your physiological ability to adapt to stress. Better adaptation during demanding days allows you to keep your focus on the innate needs of your body.

2

THE SCIENCE

"All scientific disciplines, Chiropractic, physics, chemistry, biology, psychology, etc., have basic and applied aspects. Basics science is more basic in the sense that without discovery of PRINCIPLES... there is nothing to apply. Applied science relies on and could not exist without basic science. For example, aviation uses two basic laws, the law of gravity and the law of aerodynamics and applies it to its objective which is flying. In the same way, Chiropractic uses two basic laws, the law of organization (universal intelligence) and the law of ACTIVE organization (innate intelligence) and applies its objective which is to locate, analyze and facilitate the correction of vertebral subluxations for the full express of the innate forces of the innate intelligence of the body."

- Claude Lessard, DC

| 3 |

QUALITY OF LIFE

"Life, or living matter, or matter-action at normal rate of speed is because of a continuity flow of energy through a continuity of matter. Break the continuity of matter, or continuity of energy, and you break the continuity of action with its consequent reduction in product and by-products."

- B.J. Palmer

PROACTIVE APPROACH

Do you believe that how you feel relates to your quality of life or how well you are functioning? The common belief is that when your body has no signs of pain or symptoms, all is well. The problem with judging how the body is functioning based on feeling, is that feeling can be a poor yardstick to measure your quality of life.

Health has been defined as "a state of complete physical, mental, and social well-being and not merely the absence of disease or symptoms." How well your body functions is based on more than the absence of disease or symptoms!

Your body has trillions of cells within it and your perception of how those cells and tissues are doing are almost nonexistent when it comes to determining how well they are functioning. Your liver is an extremely important organ in your body as it helps your body digest food, store energy and get rid of poisons and toxins. So if it's an important organ, shouldn't you have awareness on how it's functioning?

If I asked you how well your liver is functioning right now you would have no idea based on pure perception or thought. You would have to go to the lab and get blood drawn for an analysis to determine what levels your proteins, enzymes and chemical substances are at. This analysis would be a much more accurate way to determine how your liver is functioning than your own feelings. If we can't determine how well we're functioning based on how we feel and we don't want to go to the lab to get blood drawn on a regular basis, what's the next best approach?

LET'S CHANGE OUR APPROACH FROM DEFENSE TO OFFENSE IN THE REALM OF TAKING CARE OF THE WELL-BEING WITHIN US AND CHOOSE A PROACTIVE APPROACH TO INVESTING INTO OUR QUALITY OF LIFE.

A defensive approach to our well-being routine is to wait until our physiology breaks down and impacts our daily life, then seek a course of action to correct the damage. An offensive approach to our well-being routine is not waiting until compensation is noticed, but rather making proactive choices that will increase our quality of life by causing more inner potential to be enhanced. Achieving optimal well-being by causing more inner potential to be enhanced is an ongoing process, which means we must constantly water the garden in order for the vegetation to thrive.

Everyone knows what to do when they enter a dark room. You turn on the lights so you can see! When the light turns on, it takes away the darkness in an instant. Darkness is the exact opposite of lightness-the two fall on opposite spectrums. The perception of the spectrum of visible light is a universal principle as it works the same in all locations with all people regardless of who you are or where you're from. Darkness is interesting in the realm of physics as it's actually the absence of the entity light. Entities and non-entities are around us all the time and for most of us we just don't give it enough recognition to care which is which.

For example, darkness is nothing-non-entity and light is the something-entity. Darkness is only present when light is absent. When you turn the light on, the photos from the light take over the location and drive the emptiness of the darkness. Another way of looking at it is the presence of light takes over the absence of light-darkness be the absence of light. The manifestation of darkness is only perceivable with the absence of light. When looking at well-being and the overall function of the body-how alive you are is the entity and how much closer you are to infirmity is the non-entity. Health is a state of complete physical, mental, and social well-being; not the absence of symptoms.

This definition is important when it comes to understanding that health or function is the entity and disease, or infirmity is the non-entity. When your body is unhealthy or sick it's due to an absence of health, or function.

For greater clarification on this point; disease or infirmity is nothing, the non-entity and health or function is the something-entity. Disease or infirmity is present when health or function is absent. When you heal or create new cells, tissues and overall well-being through the recuperative power of the body to maintain coordinated function, the coordinated function within the body takes over the location and drives the emptiness of the disease or infirmity out of the body. Another way of looking at it is the presence of health or function takes over the absence of disease or infirmity-sickness is the absence of well-being. The manifestation of disease or sickness is only perceivable with the absence of health or normal function.

FUNCTIONAL EFFICIENCY

The modern consensus in the Chiropractic profession is that well-being is not related to the absence of symptoms, it's correlated to levels of functional efficiency. Functional efficiency as the context of how your body operates as the entity. Functional efficiency within your body is the entity and the presence of disease or infirmity is the non-entity.

Entity is a scientific word used to describe what's actually in existence. The non-entity is a sign that that entity is no longer in existence. Let's look at a couple examples so you can get a better understanding on how to raise your quality of life. Heat vs. cold is a great example of entity vs. non-entity. Can you guess which one is the entity and which one is the non-entity? You're correct if you said heat is the entity! You cannot create a non-entity, so that means you cannot create cold. Cold is only present when you remove heat from existence. Your refrigerator or air conditioner do not create a cold environment, they merely remove heat from the location. Light vs. darkness can be our follow-up example to describe in detail the case of entity vs. non-entity. Let's try it again, which one is the entity and which one is the non-entity? You're correct again if you said light is the entity! If you went outside during the day, the only way to create darkness is by blocking the lightness. Health, well-being, function, or quality of life within your body is the entity, and disease or infirmity being is the non-entity. Function and well-being is your normal state and you only can produce disease or infirmity if you take function or well-being away or block it from being present.

So how do you raise your quality of life? Chiropractic acknowledges the relationship between the innate recuperative power of the body to recuperate when structural integrity is optimal. Quality of life is related to functional efficiency and functional efficiency is related to structural integrity. Function is related to structure due to the complementary properties. Structure can be viewed in more detail as the form, characteristics and particular condition or state of something. Function is the ability to operate in a proper, or particular way due to the qualities of the structure.

You can raise your quality of life when your structure has normal qualities! To illustrate, balls are structurally round and bounce when they're inflated to the proper form. When you deflate the ball the structure and characteristics change-it no longer bounces and it's no longer round. Round structure produces a bouncing function.

How is your body functioning? Most if not all of us cannot answer that question with one-hundred percent certainty.

For instance, you could feel fine today and die tomorrow from a severe heart attack. The heart attack is the first and last sign of disease or infirmity. If you asked someone right before they were to experience this life shortening heart attack "how is your body functioning?" Chances are they would reply back, "great, I feel fine." But, inside their heart lacks proper or normal structural integrity which is therefore interfering with proper function leading to a lower quality of life. As this case example demonstrates, we cannot and should not determine how well our body is functioning based on how we feel. If we cannot look at how we feel as a valid indicator of how well we are functioning-how do we know how much functional integrity we hold within our body? In order to answer that question, let's define structure first.

Structure is defined as a noun as "the arrangement of and relations between the parts or elements of something complex." Structure is defined as a verb as "a construct or arrangement according to a plan."

I would like to relate structural integrity within the body as a noun and a verb due to the fact that we are human beings, human as the noun and being as the verb. In that case, structural integrity within our human body is the arrangement of our atoms, cells, tissues, and organs in relation to each other to form the complex organism according to the plan to produce function, well-being or optimal quality of life. That's a mouthful, but the simple way of describing structural integrity and functional efficiency is with one word-coordination. The coordination of all the atoms, cells, tissues and organs working together for the greater good of being alive! Let's turn our attention to coordination and how it relates to raising your quality of life.

So how do you experience better coordination from within? Before we get ahead of ourselves, let's focus on how coordination takes place. If there are trillions of cells in the body all working in an organized state, there needs to be a system that can handle that much information without getting bogged down by receiving and sending orders from that many cells.

Your coordination is directed from the functions of the neurological system. Your neurology consists of the brain and its billions of neurons, the spinal cord as an extension of the brain and the nerves that branch out from the spinal cord that physically or chemically connect with every cell in the body. Your neurological system is one of the earliest systems to develop in embryological growth, last to be developed and is currently recognized as the last system to be physiologically working before death is pronounced. The beginning stages of neurological development begins with a tube of nerves forming, that separate out into the brain, spinal cord and peripheral nerves that have tiny buds connected at the ends. As the embryo develops the complexity of the neurological system increases and so do the buds that are connected at the end the nerves. These buds turn into the glands and organs that make up our body such as the heart, stomach, intestines, adrenals, thyroid gland and so on. All of the embryological development that takes place is similar to an apple seed that sprouts out the first branch that turns into many with apples connected at the end of the branches. The seed being similar to the neurological system and the apples being similar to our internal glands and organs.

If you've ever gone to an apple farm during the fall to pick the best apples that nature has developed you'll notice a trend with the quality of fruit being grown. The apples that are mushy and barely surviving come from trees that are not functioning well with cracks and holes in the bark or branches that are not healthy or even dead. The apples that are ripe and crisp come from trees that have healthy bark and strong branches. Apple farmers realize that the fruit is identified by the tree;

fruit will be good if the tree is good and fruit will be bad if the tree is bad. This makes sense, right? Well, coordination and functional efficiency (entity) rely upon the neurological system (ie. branches) to connect to all parts of the body (ie. apples) to work in a coordinated state.

IF FUNCTIONAL EFFICIENCY IS THE DOOR TO RAISING YOUR QUALITY OF LIFE, COORDINATION IS THE KEY TO OPEN THAT DOOR.

Coordination in your body is when all the trillions of cells are working together in relationship to ensure overall harmony. When you look at companies, athletic teams or bands, and they're beating to the rhythm of one drum or coordinating together and the outcome is harmony or productivity. This concept of coordination and function as the entity is vital to grasp in order to know logically how to raise your quality of life. Coordination within your body is the organization of the complexity of the trillions of cells to smoothly and efficiently work together.

Coordination in general within the body is an automatic or unconscious process. You can't will yourself, besides breathing and moving, to coordinate more. But you do have the ability to ensure coordination is working optimally within your body through structural integrity of the system that directs coordination-the neurological system. The coordinating necessities of life are all impacted directly by the neurological system through physical or chemical connection with every cell in the body.

Your adrenal glands automatically or unconsciously are hormones (adrenaline and steroids, aldosterone and cortisol) producing organs that make chemicals that are vital to life. The adrenal glands are located directly above your kidneys and have the purpose to produce chemicals that help regulate blood pressure and sugar levels, metabolism and reaction to stressors.

Adrenaline affects your neurological system and is part of the fight or flight response. This sympathetic neurological response is activated when stress is high and or your body's physical demands outweigh the rest and recovery necessary for the parasympathetic neurological response to occur. Cortisol increases blood glucose levels and is an antagonist against insulin so glucose stays in the blood and can be metabolized from stored fat for energy. Aldosterone helps regulate sodium and potassium levels, which helps control blood pressure and electrolytes in the blood. These adrenal gland chemicals that play a vital role in your day to day function need to be at perfect balance and for the coordination of blood pressure, blood sugar levels and fight or flight response to occur.

Your body's Innate Intelligence utilizes the neurological system to communicate back and forth between the adrenal glands and brain for the right chemical to be produced at the right time with proper quantity. The adrenal glands are neurologically connected to your spinal cord through nerves that exit out your spine at the T9, T10, T11 and T12 region.

What's the purpose of knowing about the adrenal glands and that your nerves are connected to your adrenal glands? This knowledge about the adrenal glands shows how intricate and vital the neurological system is in the autonomic day to day functions to produce well-being or normal function. "Function" can be defined as an activity or purpose natural to or intended for a person or thing. Our body has an Innate Intelligence that is the self healing principle that organizes natural "Function" within us and it's coordinated through the neurological system.

Your neurological system can affect the function of every part of the body by coordinating the tissues and organs the nerve is innervated with. The spinal bones house and protect the nerves traveling to your internal organs so the brain can properly coordinate function of the tissues and organs. If spinal integrity is less than optimal, organs and tissues can be negatively affected.

Dysfunction in the spine can affect the entire body's well-being due to the following principle: In order for the whole to be 100%, the parts making up the whole need to be 100%.

This principle of wholeness in the body and everything affecting everything can be related to an analogy of water in a bucket. Joseph

Strauss, DC in his 1996 *"Enhance Your Life Experience"* describes how adding to the bucket can enhance your quality of life. He states, "If we cannot know what is normal for our body, how can we work toward maximum health and know we are moving in the right direction?"

Building off the analogy that Joseph Strauss described with adding to the bucket, Imagine your well-being like a bucket 100% full of water. Everyone has different body structures, sizes and capacity to house and maintain the water. Your well-being or wholeness is the water that is housed inside your bucket. Your body strives for 100% fullness or optimal well-being with both an inborn recuperative power to refill the water.

You don't have to do anything to promote this innate power to heal, it's a natural, inborn faucet that fills the bucket full of water. The faucet does have a handle on the influences of the flow of water, and that faucet is the positive choices you make. These choices of well-being replenish your body and fill your bucket to the top every night when you sleep. When you choose to be proactive in filling your bucket, it can be in the form of things like eating well, getting adequate exercise and rest, or having a positive mental attitude. Your choices determine the pressure of water flow of the faucet.

When you do this, your bucket will move toward fullness due to a steady flow of water that comes from the faucet. However, there's a problem with our well-being bucket: it leaks! When you choose to do less than what's necessary to fill your bucket, the contents within your bucket may lower due to life's demands and stressors. The faucet may still be dripping, but the pressure of the water flow is not as strong as it could be to keep your bucket full. Your bucket may leak at the rate at which your proactive choices overflow the bucket when it becomes full, or at the rate stressors exceed the replenishing drip from the faucet. Now your bucket is less than full and when water levels get low, dysfunction can occur within the contents of the bucket. The bucket, when low on water now becomes affected by the environment it's surrounded by. This environment poses a natural stressor on the bucket and the first attempt at breaking the bucket down, is in the form of rust.

Rust happens when the alloys of the bucket mix with the oxygen and leftover water. When filled with enough water, this reaction could not complete its damaging process . Now the rust turns this healthy bucket into a weak bucket with a slow erosion of holes beginning to occur. If only we would have known that that bucket was less than 100% full for the past several years that it takes for this chemical reaction to occur. There were very few warning signs that the bucket was only half full.

The key is to keep replenishing or adding water to the bucket before signs that the water level is low. Waiting until we are thirsty to drink water is a reactive approach that can create rust in the bucket.. When you feel thirsty, it's a sign that you're already dehydrated. Similarly, don't wait for your bucket to be low on well-being before you ensure your faucet is refilling to its capacity. When the levels of well-being are low in your bucket, it lowers your ability to adapt to life's stress.

Choosing the right well-being habits to keep the faucet on high replenish mode. The ability to have a healthy bucket to hold the contents of the water. Finally, the ability to have a healthy faucet. The faucet is often overlooked because it's part of the bucket and water, but is not as visible as the bucket or water. The faucet hides from everyday eyes, but when you look closely you can see the posture of the faucet and the overall function of the faucet. The faucet is similar to the spine within our body. The spine is the highway of neurological impulses that flow from the brain to the body. The brain being the water supply to the city or well and the body being the bucket. The spine also has handles in the form of little bones that can rotate and shift from the right to the left or left to right and even forward and backwards. These handles can positively or negatively influence the flow of neurological impulses in the way of protecting or interfering through the intimate relationship of structure and function of the spinal anatomy and neurological tissue.

The Adjustment Advantage is concerned with the integrity of the spinal joints that structurally house and protect the neurological system between the brain and the body. The Adjustment Advantage can help restore proper structural relationship within the spinal joints which allows your body's innate recuperative forces to function in harmony and allow all the handles to be open so the water contents can be in full replenish mode. This can help keep your faucet in the refilling process of your bucket. You don't have to understand all the factors or how the cause-effects relationship works in order to know that including positive elements in your way of living can contribute to a higher quality of function.

Your quality of life is a complexity of physical, mental and psychological states combined to create an overall state of well-being. The three dimensions of your quality of life are interconnected through the neurological system and must be balanced to live optimally. If your neurological system is malfunctioning due to interference, your ability to reach your desired potential can be lessened. Your quality of life is a complexity of trillions of reactions with trillions of causes and effects taking place within your body. You can create a higher state of well-being by simply introducing positive elements that contribute to the balance of these reactions.

ABOVE-DOWN-INSIDE-OUT COORDINATION

Realizing that well-being is what is in existence, and disease or infirmity is only present when well-being is missing is the next step towards making a small alteration a higher potential towards wholeness. When you understand the basic principle of how well-being is produced, you'll be more likely to make decisions to keep the light on in order to chase out the darkness.

Chiropractors have a long standing acronym that was developed in the early 1900's when B.J. Palmer was developing the profession through his family's school Palmer Chiropractic in Davenport Iowa. The acronym is "ADIO" which stands for Above-Down, Inside-Out.

ADIO is a principle that applies to how the body functions in a complete state of well-being. The meaning is that the brain is the control and coordinating center of the body that is "Above" the rest of you. The control and coordination from "Above-Down" travels through your neurological system on the "Inside" of your body to the "Outside" through mental impulses. The Above-Down, Inside-Out process of coordination and control of the trillions of cells and their respected tissues, glands and organs for the overall complete state of function and well-being is a principle that breaks down and simplifies the complex processes of physiology and body function. When complete function and well-being were just developing within your body when you were an embryo, the first organ to develop ahead of the rest of the body was your neurological system. The brain and its spinal cord extended out throughout your entire body and connected to every major organ that was in the process of being created from your original two cells. These vital connections taking place during the first couple weeks of your gestation created a pathway of coordination and control for your body to function in a state of harmony and coordination.

Wholeness is vital for the trillions of cells to cooperate and not compete against each other. The trillions of cells are similar to the old saying that branches on a tree are intelligent enough not to compete with each other, but rather branch out towards the sun to help the overall survival of the tree. Our body is neurologically connected together and coordinated and controlled via the brain, spinal cord and nerve roots extending from Above-Down, Inside-Out, similar to the seed sprouting its first root upward towards the sky with branches and fruit intimately connected to the source of its first expansion.

Our internal biochemistry directly impacts all levels of human physiology and our quality of life. Our biochemistry can be one of the greatest contributors to how our body functions. Trillions of internal chemical reactions are functioning within the body in order for health to be present. When your internal biochemistry is in harmony and balance, you demonstrate wholeness or well-being.

Imbalances or malfunctioning in the proper pathways of chemical actions results in less wholeness and well-being. Chemical structure relates to function, with each chemical having a specific structure for purpose and function.

Examples in the following for how chemicals influence our bodily functions. State of mind, energy levels and coordination can all be enhanced or altered through specific chemicals that change the internal biochemistry composition within the body. State of mind can be enhanced through specific chemicals such as: endorphin, oxytocin, serotonin and dopamine which are feel good chemicals produced through your neurological system. Energy levels can be enhanced with a chemical called caffeine which is a neurological stimulant that gives your physiology a boost. Coordination can be altered through a chemical called alcohol which can decrease function of the neurological system in regards to proper balance, hand-eye coordination and reaction time.

Chemicals either injected or created from within glands and tissues are directly influencing your body's ability to perform on all levels. Your body is chemically structured from atoms of elements that combine to form the molecules that make up the cells, tissues, organs, systems and the organism as a whole. This level of structure forms the backbone of our Above-Down, Inside-Out principle to how the body functions in a complete state of well-being. The Above-Down, Inside-Out level of organization for chemical structure relating to function is as follows:

1. Cells: Cells are the smallest unit in the body, so it's the most inner aspect of your physiological processes associated with your health and well-being. Your cells are made up of the specific chemical components that can accomplish specific purposes and functions within the body.

2. Tissues: Tissues are composed cells with similar chemical components that collectively can work together to accomplish a shared purpose and function within the body. Examples of tissue

type are; epithelial tissue, connective tissues, muscle tissue and neurological tissue.

3. Organs: Organs are when you combine two or more tissues together to perform a shared specific purpose and function within the body. An example for an organ is the heart that includes epithelial tissue, connective tissue, muscle tissue and neurological tissue creating one organ.

4. Systems: Systems are when you combine organs together to perform a specific purpose and function within the body. An example of this would be the digestive system combining the salivary glands, pharynx, esophagus, stomach, small intestine, large intestine, liver, gallbladder, pancreas and rectum.

5. Organism: Your entire body is one organism controlled and coordinated from Above-Down through the neurological system sending messages through the nerves for specific chemicals to be produced and actions and reactions to occur within the trillion of cells that make up the tissues, organs and systems within the body from the Inside-Out to sustain well-being or physiological life as we call it.

Within each of us resides an Innate Intelligence that coordinates your ability to function through a balanced biochemistry. This innate power guides the chemical processes of your body described above for overall well-being and balance. Your Educated Intelligence also aids in the proper choices in what to eat, how much to exercise and when to go to sleep, but is only aiding the innate power that coordinates the trillions of cells for chemical actions. Together, the choices you're making for your well-being and your Innate Intelligence keep the trillions of cells functioning in a state of coordination creating a balance of inner biochemistry.

Your Innate Intelligence of the body utilizes your brain to control and coordinate "Above-Down" through your neurological system to every cell, tissue, organ and system "Inside-Out" of your body via mental impulses to keep your biochemistry balanced. The Above-Down,

Inside-Out principle signifies coordination and balance from the in-side-out. It's purpose is to take the complex physiological actions within the trillions of cells, tissues and organs and simplify the processes. This form of reasoning is useful for our ability to learn how to work with our body to increase our quality of life.

Raising our quality of function is always a matter of how much harmony is within us. Harmony and balance is a chemical orchestra within us. The common term for this harmony is homeostasis. Our internal biochemistry harmony directly impacts all levels of your human physiology, performance and quality of life. Within every thought, action or reaction comes with an intricate balance of chemical production to create a symphony of physiological effects. The physiology in your body has a cause-effect relationship as it relates to proper and improper function. Similar to a light switch, when you flip the switch up it turns the light on-flip it down it turns the light off. This is a cause-effect relationship.

Your body could be compared to the room or home and when you make choices for your well-being- that's you flipping the switch up or down depending upon whether those choices are good or bad for your chemical pathways and overall biochemistry balance. Your Innate Intelligence of the body is always creating forces for flipping the switch up for more light, health and well-being. We have already discussed that the universe striving for more good or more growth as being alive is a sign that healing, homeostasis and well-being are evidence alone for this process. The biochemistry in your body demonstrates this cause-effect relationship as it relates to proper and improper function. This interrelatedness is so intricate that many times, causes may have other factors that intertwine together in the cause-effect relationship.

The problem with the cause-effect principle, as it relates to bio-chemistry or human physiology, comes down to determining what the exact cause-effect relationship is; because everything contributes to anything in physiology. Factors contribute to the cause-effect relationship. These factors create an interrelatedness so intricate that many times, causes that we know work for person A, may be different for person B as person B has other factors that create an altogether different cause-effect relationship when comparing person A and person B. Another problem with the cause-effect relationship, as it relates to human physiology is trying to determine all the unknown factors involved or influencing the known cause-effect actions or reactions in the pathways of balancing biochemistry. You could say that within your body, everything contributes to anything.

This cause-effect relationship of stress and adaptation to it impacts each of us differently. Stress has a tendency to break down your physiology in everyone when adaptation to it is less than the forces affecting the physiology, but how it breaks down your physiology is dependent upon unique factors.

If we look at two people who have the same stress filled environment, they can experience two very different effects on their bodies: one person may suffer a heart attack, while the other person may develop ulcers. Factors are a part of physiology and contribute to the cause and effect relationship of well-being and factors can create different results in the cause-effect relationship.

EVERYTHING IN YOUR BODY HAS THIS CAUSE-EFFECT RELATIONSHIP WORKING AT THE CELLULAR LEVEL, TISSUE LEVEL, ORGAN LEVEL, SYSTEMS LEVEL AND DON'T FORGET THE ORGANISM LEVEL SO OVERALL FUNCTION CAN OCCUR.

Within these five levels-you have an estimated seventy trillion cells functioning in an inter-relatedness for overall function. That means you have one long mathematical equation with over seventy trillion variables that just include the cells as the variable. If we took this conversation to a whole different level, you could open each cell up and see what's inside and create more unknown variables as each cell is a chemical producing factor creating actions and reactions.

Want to go even further? Each cell is made up of atoms and these atoms are made up of photons, electrons and neutrons that are being studied by physicists and the current science on these atoms point to a whole different theory of cause-effect relationship called quantum theory.

Quantum theory in simple terms is that the photons, electrons and other particles that make up the atoms that make up everything in the universe have characteristics to their behavior that are different and sometimes unpredictable-unique cause-effect relationships!

Going back to the question at hand, there are so many factors or variables involved with this cause-effect relationship of how your human body functions as a whole complete organism you have to leave room for unknown variables or factors. Your quality of life is a complexity of trillions of chemical reactions taking place within your body and knowing that by introducing positive factors that contribute to the balance of these reactions, overall better function can take place due to the body's innate recuperative power or Innate Intelligence striving to keep the body in a state of biochemical balance. Quality of life is a complexity of physical, mental and social states combined to create an overall state of well-being.

The three dimensions of quality of life are interconnected and must be balanced by a state of complete function from within to live optimally. Every single part of your body works in union with one another through the control and coordination of the neurological system. Because of this, many aspects of your quality of life may benefit from a better functioning body.

Knowing that the physiology in your body has a cause-effect relationship as it relates to proper and improper functions can help you make proper choices on investing into your overall well-being. When making choices that have a positive benefit for your body's Innate Intelligence, you begin to realize that simplifying your choices can make the decision making easier to work with your body. You can ask yourself, is this choice going to cause good or bad effects for your body? Making more choices for good effects influences your body to function in harmony with your body's Innate Intelligence. Making positive choices for your body to function better can pivot on the fact that your internal biochemistry balance can influence your overall health and well-being.

Here are seven chemical processes that are responsible for optimal biochemistry balance within your body that you can work with your body's Innate Intelligence from Above-Down-Inside-Out:

1. Nutrition: Nutrition is the building block for the maintenance of physiological processes inside the body and for the ability to balance your overall biochemistry, you are what you eat. What are you eating and drinking?

2. Movement: Your body gets chemically stronger through movement by boosting your overall metabolism. Are you moving your body?

3. Respiration: Respiration produces energy that is essential for the body's survival through a chemical called oxygen. Are you breathing and picking up your heart rate?

4. Excretion: Getting rid of toxic chemicals is a necessity to avoid breeding grounds for lack of health. Do you sweat and digest what you eat?

5. Growth: Physiologically speaking, you grow more when you're sleeping through a chemical called growth hormone. They say you're either growing stronger or getting weaker in the body-are you getting adequate amounts and quality of sleep?

6. Reproduction: Generating new offspring for the survival of your genome is characteristic of being alive and is a biochemistry orchestra with many different chemical pathways playing a role for increasing your chances of reproduction.

7. Responsiveness: Monitoring, detecting and responding to changes in your body's internal and external environment is a necessity of life and your neurological system is your body's primary tool for adaptation and responsiveness. Chemicals within the neurological system called neurotransmitters are creating and directing the impulses of how we act, react and even feel. Neurological impulses travel from the brain to the body and back to the brain travel through the spinal cord and nerves. The communication between the brain and body through the neurologi-

cal system directs and coordinates the body's entire biochemical equilibrium for harmony and proper function. How is your body responding and adapting to the internal and external stressors in your life?

| 4 |

FORCES

"The Chiropractic view upon health and regulation within the body is one of intellectual causation. The mental impulse is an integral component of the philosophic deduction."

- Rob Sinnott, DC, DPhCS

INNATE FORCES

The fact of the matter is, everything is energy. The desk you sit at during the day is energy, the car you drive to work is energy. The body you live in is energy. All forms of matter are energy. Nothing is solid, just different speeds of energy.

Science recognizes that everything within our universe is made out of the same atoms, and these atoms are composed of packets of energy that spin and vibrate at different levels which create the different forms of matter. In short, the energy that makes up the matter throughout the Universe is particles and subatomic particles that move as fast as light.

Light comes in different waveforms, and depending on which waveform the light is, we may or may not see it. The speed of the wave-form is what determines whether or not we can see it. If everything in this Universe is energy and within the core of all energy are particles that move as fast as light, then we have within us hidden forms of energy that cannot be seen by the eye alone.

Within us is energy that is produced through the inner recuperative power of the body via the neurological system to operate our body's trillions of cells for the purpose of communication and coordination at speeds of 119 meters per second. For comparison, light travels at finite speeds of almost 300,000,000 meters per second. Hidden within you are neurological impulses with the ability to influence the behavior of cells, tissues and organs through the power of energy or force. You have power hidden within every physical or mental impulse for the means of operating your body!

You are a walking body of potential energy, which some educated estimates say is more than what the hydrogen bomb's potential energy held to explode. Energy and mass are equal. Energy is matter being transformed, or is potential energy waiting to be transformed. Depending on how big your body is, you can take the size and plug it into Einstein's $E=mc^2$ equation to get an estimate of the amount of force of energy within you! In Chiropractic, we have the same perspective with the human body as apple farmers do with their trees and fruit.

Chiropractors realize that the cells, tissues and organs are identified by the neurological system; cells, tissues and organs will function well if the neurological system is physically and chemically able to connect to the end destination and vice versa. Cells, tissues and organs will not function well if the neurological system is in a state of dysfunction physically or chemically. All parts of our body are directly or indirectly connected to the nerves, just like apples are directly connected to the branches and indirectly to the trunk and roots of the tree. If the roots and trunk of the tree are harmed or injured, then the apples have the potential to be affected.

The apple tree and fruit analogy with the human body is a way to comprehend functional efficiency and how there is a physical connection that must be clear and free of any damage or interference for the life force to supply the end product. The ability to physically harm perfect coordination of fruit production through injury to the trunk or branches of a tree makes you comprehend the whole tree and its fruit being one organism with parts working together. The human body's ability to function toward optimal efficiency requires a healthy neurological system to supply life forces throughout the body. The nerves are one of the first cells and systems to develop in embryology and last to function before death is pronounced. 70 trillion cells coordinating together require a sound coordinating system to function in harmony and that system is the neurological system. Similarly, your computer doesn't just operate on hardware alone, it needs sound coordinating software to express the potential within it.

According to Reggie Gold's 1998 *"Philosophy of The Triune of Life."* your body requires intelligence to maintain the organization, matter to express the intelligence and force to link the two together. All three elements must be present for physiology to function in a coordinated state. Your quality of life is the expression of intelligence through matter with energy connecting the two. In order for your body to function at its highest potential, there must be 100% intelligence, matter and energy. All three elements form the components to perfect the coordination of the trillions of cells.

The Triune of Life explains the relationship between form and non-form, and the link, or force connecting them together. According to this Chiropractic theory, we can describe the human body as a three dimensional being composed of intelligence, force/energy and matter. The combination of form and non-form makes up a state of complete physical, mental and social well-being. Form being the matter and non-form being the intelligence and force/energy. The form and non-form must be connected together through force in order for functional efficiency to express well-being throughout the trillions of cells.

The topic on universal and Innate Intelligence has already been discussed, but will be briefly reviewed to comprehend how force is expressed in your living breathing body. The intelligence in our body is always one-hundred percent because it is a principle or law similar to the law of gravity. You can't take the law of gravity and make it work less than one-hundred percent of the time, it's always working. The same is true for the Innate Intelligence in our body, it's always working one-hundred percent of the time. Due to the principle of intelligence being one hundred percent efficient, the force that is generated by the principle of intelligence must also be one hundred percent efficient. The energy generated within the body is always one-hundred percent, due to the source of it coming from the Innate Intelligence. If your Innate Intelligence and innate force are always known variables that are efficiently perfect, then matter and the connection between intelligence and matter must be the weak link in the equation of well-being. Limitations of matter, or less than one-hundred percent normal function of matter, is not the focus of The Adjustment Advantage. The focus of The Adjustment Advantage is the connecting link between the form and non-form, the force being expressed through the neurological system.

Chiropractic looks at your quality of life as the representation of, and connection to, an optimal state of function; related to your overall structural integrity for the coordination of trillions of cells that make up the tissues and organs for well-being. If we're not going to discuss limitations of matter, and it's a known fact that matter is an essential element in connecting to a higher quality of life, then we must accept the fact that none of us will ever be one-hundred percent functional beings. We will always fall short due to many variables. Reggie Gold, DC has stated, "If you really want to be healthy, choose your grandparents." What he is saying is, you will always have genetic limitations (nature) embedded within you, and you will always have tendencies (nurture) of your family who raised you in circumstances out of your control. This doesn't mean you shouldn't try to change your past circumstances with better choices today and in the future. Rather it implies that who we are is in part due to who our parents are.

Connecting to a higher quality of life within the context of this book will focus on the two other elements of The Triune of Life: intelligence and force/energy. Both of these are non-form in nature, meaning that the methodology and focus will be on wholeness and well-being.

I would like to open your mind to the idea that non-form is just as vital to optimal function and well-being as is form. We just can't put our hands around intelligence or energy, we can only look at the characteristics of them.

One characteristic being the harmony that resides within us. Harmony, as in the combination of simultaneously working cells, tissues and organs. This coordination within our body is more powerful than any computer out there. There are estimates that there are over 100 billion neurons (nerve cells) per human being. They calculate that there are more neurological connections (nerves coordinating information) in the human body than stars in the galaxy. The amount of information that the neurological system can process and coordinate is millions of bits of information per second. This coordinating system is beyond comprehension. The neurological system is designed for coordination through interpreting information from the external and internal environment, and then sending information to all parts of the body to maintain a state of harmony.

Coordination is the key that opens the door to physiological efficiency. Coordination is accomplished through the body's neurological system sending and receiving information to and from the brain via the spinal cord and nerve roots, just like the apples blossoming at the end of the branches.

Chiropractic is focused on co-creating a higher state of coordination at the neurological level by locating levels of interference in the information that connects your body's Innate Intelligence with the matter that makes up the body.

THIS INFORMATION IS CONVEYED THROUGH THE NEUROLOGICAL SYSTEM AND IN CHIROPRACTIC WE REFER TO IT AS MENTAL IMPULSES.

Have you ever had the impulse to just do something? Did you do it? Impulse is both physical and non-physical. In physics, impulse is calculated by equating the amount of force over time, or how much effort or energy is being generated. This is a physical definition. In the Oxford Dictionary, impulse is defined as "a sudden strong and unreflective urge or desire to act; something that causes something to happen." The Oxford definition is non-physical. The two definitions together are necessary to comprehend how the physical and non-physical can coexist when discussing physiology, especially neurology.

The general definition of a nerve impulse in the biological world is a coded signal transmitted along a nerve through electrical means. The purpose of the nerve impulse is to relay information from point A to point B. What information is it relaying? It depends on who you ask!

All viewpoints on nerve impulses agree on how nerves relay information, but what information is being sent from origin to destination depends upon who you ask. In biology, nerves relay information that tells you how cold or hot something is, whether or not you hear a noise and if an injury was painful or not.

The five senses; taste, sight, touch, smell and sound all utilize nerve impulses to relay information to your brain. In psychology, nerves relay information about how you feel about someone, what past memories are interfering with your day to day choices, and how people ask when the neurological system is diseased.

In Chiropractic, nerve impulses also have another name: mental impulses. Mental impulses are not just electrical activity that pass through the nerve, but are electrical activity with a non-physical message embedded within the code for the purposes of coordinated activity throughout the entire body. Your physiology depends upon individual parts working together as one unit and due to the trillions of cells that need to cooperate with each other, there needs to be a system in the body that's responsible for everyone to get along. That system is your neurological system and the mental impulse is like the Morris Code, relaying the proper instructions for all cells, tissues and organs to work in harmony.

R.W. Stephenson defined mental impulse in his 1927 book "*The Chiropractic Textbook*" as: "a unit of mental force for a specific tissue cell, for a specific occasion - a special message to a tissue cell for the present instant. It differs from a universal force in that it is constructive and is for a particular moment and need of coordination, while universal forces are not constructive in particular and are for all moments, too general to be coordinative (Prin. 10,15)."

The thought that there are packets of information traveling through our neurological system to all parts of our body is astonishing. Just think, right now your brain and heart are communicating about whether or not you're sitting down or if you need to get up and run a marathon. In this case, these mental impulses relay information back to your brain so that information can be sent to your legs on how much blood is needed for your activity of either sitting or running 26.2 miles. The transmission of these mental impulses rely upon the unique make up of your neurological system.

The nerves' capability to transmit information at lightning speed is due to the cable insulated structure that can provide a pathway of electrochemical communication without interference. The bundle of nerve tracts carry a difference in electrical charge from the inside compared to the outside, similar to a battery having a plus and negative side of charge. When the nerve is ready to relay information or it's activated, there is a difference in electrical charge within the nerve due to charged atoms and molecules moving in and out of the neuron. All of this is taking place at race car speeds of 250 miles per hour!

Every cell in your body requires mental impulses at every moment. That means there are trillions of mental impulses for every moment in your body to maintain proper function throughout the body. Trillions of impulses per moment requires efficient means of communication.

One theory is that the information is sent through codes of modulation. Changes in amplitudes and frequency of electrical charge relay different information. Amplitude and frequency alterations to relay information isn't new to science. When you turn your radio on, you hear music through this same process. The modulation of amplitude and frequency is what AM and FM stands for. The amplitude and frequency can be transmitted thousands of miles away via electromagnetic waves through a process of modulation. Modulation is basically change.

Changing the amplitude and frequency of radio waves to hear the specific information being transmitted from radio tower to car or home. The theory is neurological wires in your body may transmit impulses in a similar manner to radio waves changing their wave amplitude and frequency.

The point to grasp is mental impulses are not just electrochemical impulses, but rather modulated electrochemical impulses with a message carried with it. Using the radio as our example, the radio isn't just electromagnetic waves. The radio is electromagnetic waves with either a song or news attached to the modulated waves. The message that's carried within the waves is the point to grasp. Your body is currently sending and receiving messages throughout the body through your neurological system.

How can you prove these mental forces exist? One way is looking at the placebo and nocebo effect. The placebo effect is proof that the body has innate healing characteristics through mental forces. The placebo effect is defined as, "a beneficial effect produced by a placebo drug or treatment which cannot be attributed to the properties of the placebo itself, and therefore must be due to the patient's own ability to naturally repair and heal from within without any outside factors or influence." The nocebo effect is similar to the placebo effect, but just in opposite realms. The nocebo effect is defined as, "a detrimental effect on health produced by psychological or psychosomatic factors such as negative expectations of treatment or prognosis."

Both the placebo and nocebo effect show how the body has innate self healing characteristics that can be turned off or on depending upon the person's belief. The mind-body connection in the placebo and nocebo effects shows how the neurological system plays a vital part in complex neurobiological reactions that are necessary for normal function to occur. As science continues to learn more about the human body, it's just as important to understand the why, as it is to understand the how, or what. The information or message being sent through the mental impulse, regardless of how it's being sent is the why to comprehend.

The impulse isn't just energy or electrochemical impulses being transmitted. The mental impulse carries with it a metaphysical force of intelligence for a specific cell at a specific time. An individual message to an individual circumstance. Messages that are packed with information are used in our day to day technology for purposes of viewing mental impulses from a common perspective. When you send a text message to a friend you can either type it out: "Hi John, it was great seeing you yesterday!" or send a emoji saying the same thing. Both messages aren't just just letters or symbols, they're messages with information embedded into them. The information with this example is gratitude, love, friendship and appreciation. This information is what's within the message.

UNDERSTANDING THAT INFORMATION IS CARRIED THROUGH MENTAL IMPULSES CAN BE COMPARED TO OUR BODY BEING A COMPUTER.

Computers have processors and hard drives to store and interpret code. The code that the computer programmer embedded into the hard drive is interpreted by the computer's processor and has information for you to perform functions and activities on the computer. If the computer has proper code written by the programmer, you can utilize the apps and key features of the computer to work efficiently. The information is what the code strung together on the hard drive. The computer code carries with it performance and function.

Your neurological system is similar to the hard drive and processor with electrochemical impulses modulating at different amplitudes and frequencies which creates a code within our body to relay a message packed with information for the performance of your cellular and tissue needs. Codes and information are not radical science. Although, they may have been up until the 1950's when James Watson and Francis Crick discovered that the structure of DNA carries with it instructions used in cellular growth, development and overall function. The specific structure of the DNA carried with it specific expression in information. Your genes are sequenced through specific amino acid language to set rules for the expression of cellular performance and function. When specific amino acids are in order they tell what proteins to make, and this turns into who you are. Alterations in the sequence change the output.

Mental impulses didn't hit the big screen in Hollywood like DNA did when R.W. Stephenson first wrote about it back in 1927. Metal impulses are still greatly under appreciated for what they do on a daily basis in our body's physiology. True, they don't carry with them the genetic blueprint, but they keep the physical blueprint working together, similar to a contractor working with the architect plans and subcontractors. Someone or something needs to make sure that all 70 trillion subcontractors (cells) are building the house with the right plans laid out by the architect. Otherwise, you have the plans (DNA) and you have the subcontractors (cells), but you have no coordinated activity for the overall goal of a functioning home (body).

It's fair to say that the physical body has within it at all times a non-physical state that conveys information for normal physiological function. The non-physical or metaphysical aspect of neurology is the tool the body utilizes to communicate throughout the trillions of cells, similar to the radio tower communicating with the millions of cars and homes within a metropolitan city. The physical body and the metaphysical information need each other for the expression of life. The mental impulse is the metaphysical aspect of physical neurology.

Just like the physical part of our body can get injured, so too can the non-physical. When you break a bone, your doctor will set the cast to prevent further damage to the injured bone tissue. This physical injury to the bone can be seen on an x-ray and sometimes even in the outer structure, depending upon how bad of an injury took place. Unfortunately, injury to the metaphysical component of mental impulses cannot be seen on an x-ray. Injury to the metaphysical aspect of physiology cannot be physically demonstrated, just its effects, or the body's self correcting efforts for the injury. When disturbances occur to mental impulses, you can describe it as interference due to the information that is being transmitted through the nerves. Interference in mental impulses cause dis-coordination or improper function due to their coordinating purposes throughout the body. Even though you cannot physically see interference, it can be just as traumatic to your body's well-being when left uncorrected. What causes one person to get the big idea that lies within the philosophy of Chiropractic, or someone else to walk away from it in search for something else to either replace it or add to it? Within the search for wisdom lies the investigative process of turning knowledge into actual perception. Our senses crave something that's real, something that we can taste, touch or hear. This process of turning information into reality can happen through several forms. Deductive reasoning is one of them.

Deductive reasoning is an act of reasoning that is characterized by, or based on the conclusion of particular instances from a general law or principle. You conclude a new thought based on an already accepted fact, principle, or truth. While you're investigating the philosophy, science and art of The Adjustment Advantage, utilizing deductive reasoning is a natural form of our thought process in search for truth and understanding. Using this thought process is a means of building your perception on foundations of principles or facts. Building perception on foundations of principles or facts means that we are deducing more principles or facts. Deductive reasoning draws information out of that which is already true. This makes more truth and fact within the new deduced perception. Deductive reasoning was used in our profession, starting with a major premise that cannot be denied, then logically concluding statements that must also be true by reasoning from the major premise. This process of deducing truth from a major premise was useful early on in the development of our profession while we were building certainty, but it is just as powerful now as it was over one hundred years ago.

In "The Chiropractic Textbook," Ralph Stephenson, DC presented the core principles of Chiropractic, and in the process of presenting the principles, he relied upon deductive reasoning. Ralph Stephenson, DC started with a major premise that cannot be denied before he started deducing the principles. The following 33 Chiropractic Principles are found in "*The Chiropractic Textbook,*" by Ralph Stephenson, DC:

1. The Major Premise – A Universal Intelligence is in all matter and continually gives to it all its properties and actions, thus maintaining it in existence.
2. The Chiropractic Meaning of Life – The expression of this intelligence through matter is the Chiropractic meaning of life.
3. The Union of Intelligence and Matter – Life is necessarily the union of intelligence and matter.
4. The Triune of Life – Life is a triunity having three necessary united factors, namely: Intelligence, Force and Matter.
5. The Perfection of the Triune – In order to have 100% Life, there must be 100% Intelligence, 100% Force, 100% Matter.
6. The Principle of Time – There is no process that does not require time.
7. The Amount of Intelligence in Matter – The amount of intelligence for any given amount of matter is 100%, and is always proportional to its requirements.
8. The Function of Intelligence – The function of intelligence is to create force.
9. The Amount of Force Created by Intelligence – The amount of force created by intelligence is always 100%.
10. The Function of Force – The function of force is to unite intelligence and matter.
11. The Character of Universal Forces – The forces of Universal Intelligence are manifested by physical laws; are unswerving and unadapted, and have no solicitude for the structures in which they work.
12. Interference with Transmission of Universal Forces – There can be interference with transmission of universal forces.
13. The Function of Matter – The function of matter is to express force.

14. Universal Life – Force is manifested by motion in matter; all matter has motion, therefore there is universal life in all matter.

15. No Motion without the Effort of Force – Matter can have no motion without the application of force by intelligence.

16. Intelligence in both Organic and Inorganic Matter – Universal Intelligence gives force to both organic and inorganic matter.

17. Cause and Effect – Every effect has a cause and every cause has effects.

18. Evidence of Life – The signs of life are evidence of the intelligence of life.

19. Organic Matter – The material of the body of a "living thing" is organized matter.

20. Innate Intelligence – A "living thing" has an inborn intelligence within its body, called Innate Intelligence.

21. The Mission of Innate Intelligence – The mission of Innate Intelligence is to maintain the material of the body of a "living thing" in active organization.

22. The Amount of Innate intelligence – There is 100% of Innate Intelligence in every "living thing," the requisite amount, proportional to its organization.

23. The Function of Innate Intelligence – The function of Innate Intelligence is to adapt universal forces and matter for use in the body, so that all parts of the body will have co-ordinated action for mutual benefit.

24. The Limits of Adaptation – Innate Intelligence adapts forces and matter for the body as long as it can do so without breaking a universal law, or Innate Intelligence is limited by the limitations of matter.

25. The Character of Innate Forces – The forces of Innate Intelligence never injure or destroy the structures in which they work.

26. Comparison of Universal and Innate Forces – In order to carry on the universal cycle of life, Universal forces are destructive, and Innate forces constructive, as regards structural matter.

27. The Normality of Innate Intelligence – Innate Intelligence is always normal and its function is always normal.
28. The Conductors of Innate Forces – The forces of Innate Intelligence operate through or over the nerve system in animal bodies.
29. Interference with Transmission of Innate Forces – There can be interference with the transmission of Innate forces.
30. The Causes of Dis-ease – Interference with the transmission of Innate forces causes incoordination or dis-ease.
31. Subluxations – Interference with transmission in the body is always directly or indirectly due to subluxations in the spinal column.
32. The Principle of Coordination – Coordination is the principle of harmonious action of all the parts of an organism, in fulfilling their offices and purposes.
33. The Law of Demand and Supply – The Law of Demand and Supply is existent in the body in its ideal state; wherein the "clearing house," is the brain, Innate the virtuous "banker," brain cells "clerks," and nerve cells "messengers."

These principles within Chiropractic are deduced from a major principle that cannot be denied. Deduction is reduction or subtraction of something. Deductive thinking is reducing new truth from something that is already true, — subtracting logic from current logic. How can we use this compelling way of thinking in regards to The Adjustment Advantage?

First, you can use this deductive way of thinking to reinforce your conviction for The Adjustment Advantage. It will help you create clarity behind the purpose of the Chiropractic Adjustment. In most cases and most topics, life is complicated, including the ideas and practices of Chiropractic. If you asked 100 different people what Chiropractic is, you would probably get 99 different answers due to the confusion in the communication and theories and principles that we've deduced throughout the past 100 years within our profession. I propose using this way of thinking to deduce principles that are true and tested. You can study these principles to find out something that you know has validity in practice and in communicating Chiropractic.

Second, use deductive reasoning in your way of communicating about The Adjustment Advantage. People at large think logically and would appreciate someone explaining how they can benefit from Chiropractic in a way they understand through reasoning. Sometimes within Chiropractic there is this approach to complicate the philosophy, science, and art through complex ideas that can create confusion and make the points of the conversation lost. Deductive reasoning creates clarity from principles that are true. Let's simplify The Adjustment Advantage through reasoning, or in the latin phrase "reductio ad absurdum," translated means, "reduce to absurdity." Let's remove all unnecessary verbiage and reduce The Adjustment Advantage to its simplest possible explanation. Reggie Gold, DC. helped thousands of Chiropractors communicate Chiropractic more efficiently to their communities. He was a master communicator of the principles of Chiropractic. All of the audios that were recorded of him explaining Chiropractic were so logical, you know he had spent time deducing his thoughts and theories to produce more true and tested principles in his message. He was the one who taught me to reduce to absurdity in one of his teachings. Reducing to absurdity doesn't mean you don't preserve some of the original principle. Keeping The Adjustment Advantage tied to the major premise keeps it connected to the roots within the profession. The most reduced, simplest form of communicating The Adjustment Advantage is through this simple principle that we all have a higher quality of life waiting for us to express, and it can be experienced by making small alterations or movement towards your desired potential.

Your highest quality of life is like the potential energy waiting at the top of the hill within a ball. It's waiting to be expressed into another form of energy or higher quality of life. In order to convert your current condition to a higher quality, you need to make small alterations or movements towards your desired potential and one influential way of making a small alteration is through a specific Chiropractic Adjustment to vertebrae that have been negatively affected by stress. This is reduced in logic, but let's not stop our search for truth and wisdom. Let us continue our investigation through further deducting reasoning on the philosophy, science and art of The Adjustment Advantage.

UNIVERSAL FORCES

Did you know that there is a constant war-like battle that takes place within your body and your environment? It can be thought of in terms of invasive forces vs. resistive forces. Invasive forces would be anything on the outside trying to get in and attack our harmony, or anything breaking down on the inside of us, creating weakness in our body armor and harmful damage due to a lack of normal resistance. Resistive forces are our body's defense mechanisms against stress that can turn a healthy functioning cell or tissue into an opportunity for apoptosis (cellular death) to occur, so the battle may be lost, but the war isn't over. The protective forces that the body holds within us are an electrochemical engagement with negative invasive forces.

The body is constantly striving for protection from any threat that may impact the overall well-being of the trillions of cells within the body. This unwavering ability to resist invasive forces has its limitations, but the amount of inner intelligence or wisdom born within all of us is coded for protection. You don't have to teach your body to protect you, it comes with the package. The Innate Intelligence of the body has one job: to keep your body alive and well against the threats and stress that break us down from either the outside-in, or the inside-out. Sleep well knowing that each night restoration and healing is on the top of the priority list for your body to fight another day's worth of warfare to being well. Did you know that stress confronts all ages?

Yes, even infants and babies encounter stress. Every single person on this planet encounters stress in their lives on a daily basis. Some of us are adapting to this stress, while others are compensating, and negatively losing an optimal state of well-being. Stress can negatively affect all of us at any age, during all seasons of life.

WE CAN'T ENTIRELY RID OUR LIVES FROM STRESS, BUT WE CAN BECOME MORE AWARE OF THE FACT THAT STRESS IS PART OF LIVING, AND FIND BETTER WAYS TO ADAPT SO THAT WE CAN BE STRONGER AND MORE RESILIENT TO THE DEMANDS AND OBSTACLES THAT WE ENCOUNTER DAILY.

Infants start adapting or compensating to stress starting as soon as conception begins and the embryo turns into a growing baby inside of Mother. As this infant is growing inside of Mother, the choices the mother makes can either negatively or positively affect the growing infant. These choices the mother makes can become the stressors that start the process of compensating or adapting to stress at an early age. For example, if Mother has chemical stress in her lifestyle, for example, drinking alcohol, smoking or even having the flu, the infant can be negatively impacted. If Mother has a healthy lifestyle, for example, having good nutrition, exercising, resting and visiting her chiropractor, the infant's development can flourish in a positive environment due to the decisions the mother makes.

Once the baby is born into this world, stress doesn't stop the process of trying to break down normal healthy physiology. Babies are eating, sleeping and trying to stay healthy just like us, so let's consider how stress might be negatively influencing them right before our eyes.

Every fall and winter the sun disappears. The weather gets cold and kids head back to school to share high fives and hugs that create a perfect storm for bacteria and viruses to be spread. The fact that cold and flu season affects all of us is known, the unknown factor is why some of us escape being victims. Adaptation is part of that unknown factor, and it can become the same source of your baby's ability to stay healthy not only during the cold and flu season, but especially during the first couple years of growing up as their immune system is developing. The point to consider is when adaptation to bacteria and viruses fails, and babies lose the battle to the foreign living organism, this process becomes an overall stressor on them at levels that become harmful for their overall well-being. Stress is all around us and babies are no different.

Being aware of the fact that infants, babies and children live in the same world of invasive forces vs. internal resistive forces will bring more clarity on what, how and why investing into your children's health is a necessity. Children have an amazing ability to adapt to stress, but as they age and develop, demands and expectations increase in their lives and positive proactive measures for their well-being are vital. Stress is everywhere and constantly combats with our ability to function in a normal state. Stress can overcome and break down our normal physiology into a state of dysfunction and disharmony without us even being aware of the effects. Chiropractic recognizes three categories of stress that can affect your body:

1. Emotional Stress
2. Chemical Stress
3. Physical Stress

Out of all three forms of stress, emotional stress has to be at the top for most potential effects. We all have thoughts running through our minds all day long, some estimates say we have over 70,000 thoughts per day, almost 3,000 thoughts per hour, or 50 per minute. With an average of one thought per minute running through your mind, and those thoughts carrying a powerful potential to do good or harm, the emotional toll these thoughts can cause is staggering. Thinking or experiencing negative or worrisome thoughts can impact our well-being, it's a fact. Just think about a time when you got so worried that your stomach turned over! Your thoughts can create a change in your bowel movements in moments. Think about the emotional stress children are under, facing social demands when it comes to relationships with classmates, or finding someone to sit with at lunch. Children might be under more emotional stress than adults, feeling stressed to perform well in classes, sports, or extracurricular activities. Emotional stress is there, and can be a burden on our internal well-being.

If you thought that emotional stress was one hard to visualize or see, so too are the hidden chemical stressors that are all around us. Inhaling, drinking or ingesting chemicals that can create internal damage to our well-being is another known fact. Eating a low nutrient based breakfast to start the day does the body no good. Drinking a sweet drink or snack when you get home from work or when the kids get home from school can be a chemical battle taking place within the digestive tract. Chemical stress is becoming more advertised and talked about as our health and well-being continues to suffer from the low nutrient foods and harmful additives that are commonly found within processed foods.

Being aware of chemical stress that silently affects your overall well-being from the inside out can be your way of eating an apple a day. Making smart and healthy choices about what not to put into your body is no different than choosing a healthy snack, such as an apple, to eat every day to keep the doctor away!

If it's not the thoughts we're thinking or the food and drink we're digesting, then the physical wear and tear of just getting through the day has the potential to cause dysfunction and breakdown on your body. Constant physical demands can create a negative compound effect on our well-being.

Tony Robbins has said, "We live in a box! We sleep in a box, we sit in a box, we drive to work in a box, we sit all day in a box, we drive home in a box and then we go to sleep in a box. This boxed in world that we live in doesn't mesh well with our body that is designed for movement and exercise." The physical toll of not moving enough and sitting too much all day is a real physical stressor that needs to be recognized.

ADAPTATION TO FORCES

As we become more aware of emotional, physical and chemical stressors, we want to find ways to increase our ability to adapt to it rather than compensate for it. Stress is constantly confronting our ability to function in its normal state, and due to the negative consequences stress can cause on the body's physiology, understanding how to adapt to it rather than compensate for it is vital for your ability to thrive at your peak potential.

When it comes to stress, you have two options to approach the harmful effects:

1. Lower the amount of stress.
2. Increase your resistance to stress.

If you had only one option when it comes to adapting to stress, which one would you choose, lowering the amount of stress, or increasing your resistance to it? Most would probably say lower the amount of stress, right? I would like to challenge your mindset by focusing on what you can control, and when it comes to stress, the most control you have is increasing your resistance to it.

When weight training or exercising, you never go to the gym and expect to lower the amount of weight you lift on the dumbbells or shorten the distance on the treadmill. You go to the gym to increase your resistance to what's making you stronger. This approach of increasing resistance builds muscle and strength. The same is true for adapting to stress, you want to be cautious of the amount of negative stress that's affecting your physiology, but when training for the marathon of life, increasing your resistance to it will create a stronger and more adaptable you to take on the daily demands and expectations.

Emotional, physical and chemical stressors are constantly breaking down your normal physiology and increasing your resistance to it is vital for optimal quality of living. The question you're probably asking is, if stress is so bad and we need to find ways to battle it, why can some people not do anything to increase resistance to it and still live a long life? You're right, some people can eat bacon every day, not exercise and live to one-hundred and three. Let's not aim for that lifestyle, but let's look at how your body is constantly striving for protection against negative stress. This inner ability to protect against invasive forces is within all of us: the Innate Intelligence of the body. You don't have to teach your body to protect you from stress, it comes with the package.

For the majority of us who can't live an unhealthy lifestyle and need to choose the right decisions for our body. Eating well, getting exercise and rest, and investing into our quality of life keeps the faucet adding back into the bucket of well-being. The more positive choices you make for your quality of life, the more the bucket fills. Even though there is a natural drip of water adding back into the bucket, we can aid in the process of restoration of a full bucket.

This inner process of your bucket of well-being naturally filling up and you aiding it has its limitations. Eating an apple a day or walking around the block are both excellent choices to add to your quality of life, but eating apples all day and walking around the block all day will inevitably turn into a stressor on your body.

The bucket of well-being wants to be full, but when filled past its limits of capacity, it can create stress on the bucket or body. Your bucket may only be able to hold five gallons and you're trying to force ten gallons into it. The excess of good can turn into a negative force. This balance of well-being is different for everyone and striving for greater awareness of how full your bucket of well-being is the journey and challenge we all should take to living towards an optimal quality of life. There's a problem with our bucket of well-being though, it leaks!

We already discussed how your bucket has limits on how full it can be before it starts leaking, but your bucket of well-being also leaks at the rate that stressors exceed replenishment from the faucet. The more stress you put on your bucket before the bucket can refill, the more your contents of well-being will leak out from the bottom. Too much stress, or not enough rest can create a leaky bucket. By doing less than what's necessary to keep the bucket full, the contents within may lower or become less balanced due to life's demands and stressors creating leaky holes at the bottom of the bucket. Our faucet may still be refilling well-being molecules of life, but the level of the water within the bucket does not stay full or balanced due to the demands and stress outweighing the recuperative power to keep the bucket full. Stress outweighing the innate healing that replenishes through the faucet can create a leaky bucket.

The key to keeping the bucket full of water is to keep the faucet's handles open to replenish the bucket before signs that the water level is low. For example, waiting until we are thirsty to drink water may be too late to replenish the body's necessities before a state of dysfunction sets in. When you feel thirsty, it may be a sign that you're already dehydrated. Similarly, don't wait for your bucket to be low on well-being before you ensure the faucet is refilling to its capacity. This approach to keeping the handles on open at all times is a logical approach to keeping the bucket full of water, because you know that stress is on constant attack creating holes that we're not even aware of.

When the levels of well-being are low in the bucket, it lowers the body's ability to adapt to life's demands or stress, creating more dysfunction and a lower level of water within the bucket, or lower quality of life. Depending upon the size of the bucket and its capacity, content levels will affect the bucket differently. Low levels of water or well-being in the bucket is similar to low gas levels in your car. When it's empty, your engine stops working. When it's running on fumes, you know the engine doesn't have as much power as it could. Our body works on chemicals, similar to the way a car works on gasoline. We require certain chemicals to create and maintain a level of well-being for our engine to burn them as fuel. Keeping your bucket of well-being full is a wise investment when you're constantly driving your body all day long.

Stress is constantly confronting your well-being in negative ways and it's your resilience to stress that determines your quality of life. How resilient are you to stress? The definition of resilience is, "being able to withstand or recover quickly from difficult conditions." Adapting to stress is being resilient. Being resilient supports balance in your well-being. Being complete in your physical, mental and social well-being requires an ability to adapt to stress. You can't escape stress, so quickly recovering or responding to it is in your best interest. Stress is everywhere. Physiological stress, or the stress response, is the body's reaction to a condition that poses a physical, chemical or psychological threat or challenge to your well-being. Stressors produce certain negative physiological responses within your body depending upon what type of stress you encounter and can take a toll on the body's normal state of function. For example, physical stressors like sustained or repeated activities, or bad posture, can negatively affect cellular and tissue formation. Chemical stressors like tobacco, alcohol or drugs can negatively affect biomechanical processes. Mental stressors like social or family demands can negatively affect overall mental function and performance.

Endocrinologist Hans Selye pioneered the study of stress with his research on the non-specific biological response to stressors: the stress response. Hans Selye coined the terms good stress "eustress" and bad stress "distress." Hans studied the system within our body that copes with stress, the hypothalamic-pituitary-adrenal axis (HPA axis). The HPA axis is our body's central stress response system.

The HPA axis is a neuroendocrine process of adapting to stress. When stressors trigger the HPA axis, hormones are triggered to signal that the threat requires the body to create biochemical changes to adapt to the stressors. The HPA axis is our body's natural inborn adaptor to negative stressors. The body can intelligently produce the right chemical at the right amount and right time to reduce stress. This can happen when the neuroendocrine process of adapting to stress is functioning optimally. Hans Selye recognized the recuperative power within the body to convert negative stress into positive normal function when adaptation is optimal within the body.

The power within your body to heal back to an optimal physiological state, or to keep the bucket full of water, increases your adaptability to stress. The more water in your bucket, the better you can adapt to life's stressors. The water level within your bucket can be enhanced through the positive choices you make. The positive choices are similar to turning the faucet handle that controls the inborn recuperative healing power for more water on or off. These positive lifestyle factors can turn the faucet on to provide more power to replenish the constant drip to a steady stream which replenishes your child's body and fills their bucket. When you choose to be proactive in filling your bucket of well-being, it can create an opportunity to be overflowing, full of water, with an abundance of balanced biochemical processes that create an effective way to increase resistance to stress. Practicing proactive lifestyle choices keeps the faucet handles on full throttle, moving the bucket of well-being towards fullness. A full bucket of well-being adapts to the ebbs and flows of stress and demands. Proactive choices determine the pressure of water flow of the faucet.

Even though we have the power to adapt to stress, that doesn't mean we win the battle every time. Stress can negatively affect anyone at any age. Too much stress and not enough resilience or adaptation to it can break down our normal physiology into a state of dysfunction and disharmony without us even being aware of the effects.

STRESS IS EVERYWHERE AND CONSTANTLY COMBATS WITH OUR BODY'S ABILITY TO FUNCTION IN A NORMAL STATE, INCLUDING THE SPINAL INTEGRITY.

Your neurological system is the primary tool for adaptation and responsiveness. Adaptation is a known biological indicator of the quality of life that remains within the organism. The Adjustment Advantage has a positive influence for your quality of life due to this intimate connection between the neurological system and adaptation and responsiveness.

Your neurological system is a powerful network of nerves that have more potential for coordination and control than any computer. Your neurological system is the connecting link between where you are now in your quality of life and the next level to better function. The neurological system coordinates all the major systems within the body such as cardiovascular, breathing and digestion.

Knowing how pivotal the neurological system is within the body for overall function should make you consciously find ways to invest into protecting this key pathway for inner biochemistry balance, responsiveness and overall adaptation to our environment. You're probably asking right now, how can I make choices to protect and invest into my neurological system? There are many choices you can make that will have positive effects on your neurological system, one choice that Chiropractors are adamant about that can have an influential impact on your quality of life is the structure-function relationship that is composed of your spinal structure and your neurological system function.

The structure of the spinal column that surrounds and protects the brain stem, spinal cord and nerves, impacts the overall function and performance of the neurological system. Your quality of the spinal structure can and does contribute towards a positive functional effect of the neurological system to coordinate and control the trillions of chemical pathways and systems throughout your body.

Your spinal structure influences the function of the neurological system which in turn influences your biochemistry and overall physiology. Function can be defined as an activity or purpose natural to or intended for a person or thing. The body's Innate Intelligence that allows self healing and coordination to be our natural state of function within us utilizes the neurological system as the primary tool for a state of optimal function to occur. Spinal integrity can influence the body to function at its peak potential due to the relationship between structure and function that is coordinated by the neurological system. When our body functions at its peak potential due to optimal spinal integrity, our quality of life can be enhanced and the trillions of biochemical actions and reactions are functioning in a state of coordination and responsiveness.

How can you better adapt to stress? One way to be more resilient is by becoming better. Better as in a more excellent quality of life physically, mentally and socially. Having a better quality of life physically, mentally and socially allows you to adapt to stress more effectively, which can create more resilience. Here are five ways to becoming better at adapting to the forces or stress in your life:

1. Rest/Recovery: Pay attention to the amount your body gets each night, this is when the body's physiology recovers from daily wear and tear.

2. Eating/Nutrition: Proper nutrition and adequate water are the building blocks for the trillions of cells that form the tissues and organs that make up our body. This is a simple but profound way to build up an armor to the day to day demands.

3. Movement/Exercise: Movement is life. Find time to create more movement in your day. Stand more, get off the couch and turn off the television. Walk more, take a daily walk around the block in the morning or before bed. Movement and engagement in sports and activities can help get us mentally and physically stronger.

4. Thoughts/Attitude: Adding to your quality of life through a positive mental attitude is a force that is just being recognized as a foundation for well-being. Just the opposite of a positive attitude is a negative attitude, which can be stress in and of itself. For example, put a negative scary thought into your mind right now and watch your stomach turn over and produce negative harmful imbalance in your biochemistry within. Positive and healthy thoughts and affirmations can be a natural way of thinking that will add to the foundation of increasing your resistance to stress.

5. Adaptability/Responsiveness: The body's ability to adapt or respond to stress is primarily through the neurological system. Neurological integrity is an integral part of the body's ability to coordinate stressors on the body. Neurological impulses travel at hundreds of feet per second for the proper responsiveness to

stress. Because the neurological system coordinates every cell and organ in your body, Chiropractor's focus on the structure of the spine being properly aligned. If spinal integrity interferes with neurological function due to misaligned vertebrae, this is termed vertebral subluxation and will be discussed in greater detail in the following chapter. The Adjustment Advantage can help increase your resistance to stress as it can strengthen the body's inherent ability to adapt to negative stress by removing neurological interference due to the structure-function relationship at the spinal cord level that vertebral subluxation influences.

| 5 |

VERTEBRAL SUBLUXATION

"Vertebral subluxation is a condition of a vertebra that has lost its proper juxtaposition with the one above or the one below or both; to an extent less than luxation; which occludes an opening, impinges nerves and interferes with the transmission of mental impulses."

- R.W. Stephenson, DC

WHAT IS VERTEBRAL SUBLUXATION?

In order to fully grasp The Adjustment Advantage, having a complete picture of vertebral subluxation will allow you to visualize the logistics of the Chiropractic Adjustment. Understanding vertebral subluxation was an early endeavor by the developer of the Chiropractic profession, and it led many professors within the profession to articulate the definition of vertebral subluxation in Chiropractic textbooks.

In 1897, D.D. Palmer had a school and students where he taught his Chiropractic methods of palpation and adjusting of the spine in Davenport, Iowa. D.D. Palmer's discovery led him to believe that vertebrae or bones in the spine could be slightly displaced and misaligned to "incomplete luxation" and interfere with neurological function.

D.D. Palmer taught his Chiropractic Students that when these vertebrae suffered an incomplete luxation, the neurological tissue that is surrounded by the bones of the spine can have an impingement and stretching to the tissue due to the new negative structure of the vertebrae in their luxated position. The Chiropractic Luxation was the founding terminology by D.D. Palmer for what we now call Vertebral subluxation.

In 1927, R.W. Stephenson's Chiropractic Textbook brought more clarity to D.D. Palmer's discovery on Vertebral subluxation. R.W. Stephenson defined vertebral subluxation in his 1927 book *"The Chiropractic Textbook"* as:

"Vertebral subluxation is a condition of a vertebra that has lost its proper juxtaposition with the one above or the one below or both; to an extent less than luxation; which occludes an opening, impinges nerves and interferes with the transmission of mental impulses."

Reviewing the R.W. Stephenson's definition of vertebral subluxation by breaking the definition down into the following elements:

1. Vertebral subluxation is a condition of a vertebra that has lost its proper juxtaposition with the one above or the one below or both; to an extent less than luxation.
2. Vertebral subluxation occludes an opening.
3. Vertebral subluxation impinges nerves and interferes with the transmission of mental impulses.

Vertebral subluxation is a condition of a vertebra that has lost its proper juxtaposition with the one above or the one below or both; To an extent less than luxation. If you break this first element to Stephenson's Subluxation Criteria down even further, you'll see that vertebral subluxation requires a vertebra in relationship with the bone above and or below, displaced or misaligned.

The spinal column is designed to protect and direct the neurological system. Starting at the top of the spine is the cranium. The cranium is otherwise known as the skull. It's there to protect the brain which is the body's headquarters for staying alive and functioning as one harmonious system. At the bottom of the cranium is a hole where the brain extends down the spine through the inside of the vertebral column.

The vertebral column is composed of 24 bones stacked on top of each other. These vertebrae are tightly knit together with soft tissue ligaments, and muscles keeping the bones articulating in proportion to just enough movement, but not too much. For most consumers of Chiropractic, this is as far to the definition of Chiropractic that has been taught. This is not a bad place to start, but when left alone without the other two elements to Stephenson's Criteria, the subluxation is downgraded in its severity to the negative effects it can have on the body as a misalignment that isn't moving properly, and needs to be repositioned for better movement and articulation. Malposition or displacement is a foundational element to Vertebral subluxation, but alone it's just that. Vertebral subluxation is more than a misalignment. Let's discuss the second element to Stephenson's Criteria to Subluxation; the occlusion to an opening.

Vertebral subluxation occludes an opening.

With the headquarters to optimal function being placed on top of your spine, the communication needs to travel through your spine in order to direct and coordinate the trillions of cells located predominantly below the head. Within each of those 24 bones within the spine is one to three openings where the neurological system can enter and exit for communication to take place between the brain and body. This communication flows through the nerves and the nerves flow through the vertebral column.

A mentor of mine would describe the architecture of the vertebral column similar to 24 donuts stacked on top of each other with the center of the donuts being the neurological system. This description is good for one out of the three openings that the vertebral column creates: the neural canal. This canal is in the middle of the vertebral column and houses the spinal cord. At the top of each vertebrae and the bottom of the adjacent vertebrae are two more openings that are produced through articulation of the vertebrae. These openings are referred to as intervertebral foramina. These openings protect the nerve roots that extend out from the spinal cord and innervate the trillions of cells throughout the body. Openings within the spinal column are directly influenced by the position and integrity of the vertebrae. If one vertebrae becomes displaced, or malpositioned compared to the one above or below, the opening that houses the nerve roots, or spinal cord can be negatively affected by creating tension from the enlarged foramina creating a state of occlusion. D.D. Palmer stated in his early writings:

"Tension, more or less than normal, causes an increase or decrease of vibration, which means a greater or less force of an impulse and a corresponding amount of heat. Nerves are never pinched or impinged upon in the foramina. Foramina are never narrowed. We do not adjust the vertebra. The vertebra itself, so far as a chiropractor knows, is never displaced, dislocated or subluxated. Any extreme movement of the articular surfaces enlarges the foramen or foramina, causing the nerves and blood vessels to become stretched and irritated, increasing its carrying power. Nerves are never shut off by the closure of the foramina. There are no dams or obstructions that restrict. Impulses are never interrupted. Reducing the lunated intervertebral articulation; diminishing the displacement of the articular processes, replacing the two articular surfaces, returns the enlarged foramen to its normal size, removes tension and irritation. Irritated nerves cause muscular contraction. The location and amount of disturbance depends upon the portion of the nervous system involved."

The first two elementals to Stephenson's Subluxation Criteria are directly related to one another and set us up for looking at the final element.

Vertebral subluxation impinges nerves and interferes with the transmission of mental impulses.

If there's too much tension on the nerve pathway, there can be interference with the communication highway and alter mental impulses. Too much tension on the nerve creates an alteration in the amplitude similar to stringing a guitar too tight and altering the musical vibration from the chords. Nerves transmit through vibrations and if the misalignment and occlusion in the neural foramina create too much tension on the nerve tissue, then this alters the message being sent via the mental impulse. You now have yourself a vertebral subluxation.

Your body is currently sending and receiving messages throughout your body via your neurological system for the purpose of uniting the inherent recuperative power, or Innate Intelligence, with all its cells, tissues, and organs. Being interference free for these mental impulses gives your inherent recuperative powers the ability to function at a higher potential. Every cell in your body requires mental impulses at every moment.   That means there are trillions of mental impulses for every moment in your body to maintain proper function. Trillions of impulses per moment require efficient means of communication.

WHAT CAUSES VERTEBRAL SUBLUXATION?

The causes of vertebral subluxation can become an information overload due to the fact that there are many different causes and many different responses to those causes based on individual adaptation. In an effort to keep the information overload to a minimum, we can simplify the specific cause of vertebral subluxation by understanding that the universe and the world we live in are governed by laws and principles. Life is governed by principles and laws that allow us to better understand either the way in which things work, or expected outcomes. For example, the law of cause and effect is that every effect has an expected cause. Every cause has an expected effect. Another law is the law of supply and demand which states that the greater the supply, the lower the demand; The lower the supply, the greater the demand.

The causes of vertebral subluxation can be understood in general through the law of supply and demand and the law of cause and effect. The law of supply and demand in relation to the cause of vertebral subluxation can be utilized to determine how the demand of stress alters the supply of physiological healing and whether there is adaptation or compensation to it. The law of cause and effect in relation to the cause of vertebral subluxation can be utilized to determine what specific causes of stress alters the physiological response of adaptation or compensation to it. Stress is everywhere and is constantly affecting our ability to function in a normal state, creating an imbalance in the law of supply and demand within.

During the middle of summer when the temperature increases and the sun and humidity takes a toll on the skin and even energy levels. The weather can be looked at as a stressor to our body's ability to function within a normal state. Too much sun and the skin can become affected. Too much heat and the trillions of cells can lose water, and dehydration can set in. This is just one example of how universal forces are everywhere and when they come in greater amounts than we can adapt to, the law of supply and demand can create new physiological states of conditions and vertebral subluxation is one of those states.

WHAT CAUSES VERTEBRAL SUBLUXATION? WHEN STRESS OUTWEIGHS THE BODY'S ABILITY TO ADAPT TO IT, VERTEBRAL SUBLUXATION CAN DEVELOP.

Chiropractors have categorized the environment of stress that can negatively affect the body into three labels: physical stress, emotional stress and chemical stress. If adaptation to one or more of these three stressors are insufficient, a perfect physiological environment for vertebral subluxation to develop occurs. In other words, when stress outweighs the body's ability to adapt to it or handle it in a manner of control, then the cells and tissues within the body can become dysfunctional. Stress vs. Adaptation. This process of stress outweighing adaptation creates a tipping point in favor of demand and alters the inner recuperative power to supply normal function.

Physical stress can be defined as external invasive forces that outweigh the internal resistive forces of the body to be in a state of balance. These external invasive forces can be major accidents or trauma, or they can be small repetitive forces that build up over time and the repetition can be too intense for the body to adapt to. These external invasive forces can cause dysfunction on the body's muscles, ligaments and vertebrae of the spine, creating an opportunity for vertebral subluxation to occur.

Chemical stress can be defined as external or internal chemicals that trigger physical reactions throughout the body, offsetting the chemical equilibrium or body chemistry balance. Chemicals within our body can be powerful agents of physiological change. For example, hormones like adrenaline, cortisol and melatonin influence health, well-being and specific physiological states of function. The body is dependent upon a state of body chemistry balance and when that balance is out of harmony, the neurological and musculoskeletal system can be affected, leading to another opportunity for vertebral subluxation to occur.

Emotional stress can be defined as internal emotional tension or mental strain that can produce physical responses throughout the body offsetting the chemical equilibrium, or physical state of balance. It's been reported that emotional stress may be the most common and most influential cause of vertebral subluxation due to the fast paced world we live in. When the body's chemical equilibrium, or physical state is out of balance due to emotional tension or mental strain, it can lead to another opportunity for vertebral subluxation to occur. Vertebral subluxation can occur in all ages and stages of life regardless of symptoms due to physical, chemical and emotional stress. Stress is real and affects all of us. Life is demanding no matter your age or state of well-being you are in. Your responsibility to take care of your body to the best of your ability includes being aware of stress and the potential for vertebral subluxation to be negatively affecting your quality of life. Regular Chiropractic Care can be a positive option to lower the opportunity for vertebral subluxation to occur and to increase your resistance towards stress and strengthen your overall function of well-being from within.

HOW DO YOU KNOW IF YOU HAVE VERTEBRAL SUBLUXATION?

How do you tell if something in your body isn't working at its normal capacity? Is it pain? Symptoms? Yes, symptomatology can be a telltale sign that something isn't right within, but in the continuum of your state of condition, symptoms are most often the last sign to show up.

Understanding how well your body functions compared to how it feels is a big step in the right direction for a higher quality of life. It's a popular belief that well-being is related to feeling good. Unfortunately, there are many people that feel fine and suffer from a lack of complete physical, mental and psychological well-being. Dental cavities, heart attacks and cancer are just a few examples of feeling good while living outside the realm of well-being. How you feel just isn't the greatest yardstick to measure how well you're functioning.

Well-being is more than just how you feel! This definition of health is important when it comes to understanding that health or function is the entity, and disease or infirmity is the non-entity. When your body is unhealthy, or sick it's due to an absence of health or function. Health is the state of complete well-being regardless of the absence of disease, or infirmity. When you heal or create new well-being through the recuperative power of the body, the well-being within the body takes over and drives the emptiness of the disease or infirmity out. Another way of looking at it is that the presence of health or function takes over the absence of disease or infirmity, and sickness is the absence of well-being.

I recommend to my clients that investing into their quality of life regardless of the absence of symptoms will produce the greatest return on investment. How do you know if you have vertebral subluxation? Using the criteria of headaches, neck pain, or back pain may not be your greatest indicator of when to see the Chiropractor due to the inconsistency of pain and dysfunction and how they correlate with each other. Dysfunction can and does occur without pain or symptoms. Vertebral subluxation does and can occur without headaches, neck pain, or back pain. So how do you know if you have vertebral subluxation if it's not solely symptomatology as a valid indicator?

CHIROPRACTORS ARE THE TRAINED PROFESSIONALS AT LOCATING, ANALYZING AND DETECTING VERTEBRAL SUBLUXATION.

The consensus within the profession is to use a multi-factor authentication approach to locate, analyze and detect vertebral subluxation. This process is similar to providing two or more pieces of evidence to verify your identity to gain access to an app or website. The Chiropractor's Multi-Factor Authentication of vertebral subluxation can be best understood by seeing the consistent 3-4 variables involved with vertebral subluxation.

The first factor in the Chiropractor's multi-factor authentication of vertebral subluxation is asymmetry. Asymmetry can be located, analyzed and detected regionally within the spine or segmentally.

The second factor in the Chiropractor's multi-factor authentication of vertebral subluxation is a range of motion abnormality. Abnormal range of motion can be located, analyzed and detected regionally within the spine or segmentally. Abnormal range of motion within the spine can be observed through active range of motion or palpated by the Chiropractor through passive range of motion.

The third factor in the Chiropractor's multi-factor authentication of vertebral subluxation is tissue, or tone alteration. Alteration in the tone of soft tissue (such as muscles, ligaments and tendons, or skin) can be located, analyzed and detected regionally within the spine and segmentally. Alteration with tone is a direct correlation with alteration with neurological expression through the tissue. When the Chiropractor detects this factor in analyzing for vertebral subluxation, it correlates with segmental joint innervation.

The fourth factor in the Chiropractor's multi-factor authentication of vertebral subluxation is somatic sensation or perception of actual, or potential tissue damage through tenderness, discomfort, or pain. Somatic sensation, or perception of injury most often is expressed through subjective communication by the person who is receiving the evaluation for vertebral subluxation. The Chiropractor's Multi-Factor Authentication of vertebral subluxation are indicators related to your ability to adapt to stress and the law of demand and supply that's taking place within your physiology.

Supply and demand is a principle of healing within the body and is in constant flux and stability based on the body's inner wisdom to keep the trillions of cells within you working together through coordination and well-being. If your quality of life is not keeping up with the demands you're placing on your body, integrate ways to create healthier habits that promote vitality, well-being and healing. Supplying your body with simple and smart choices that promote health, healing and well-being can give you a competitive advantage for the demands on keeping your quality of life in equilibrium. Life is demanding, and due to the negative effects life's demands have on the body it's your responsibility to take care of your body to the best of your ability. These negative effects or stressors from the demands of life are present no matter what age you are, even for kids.

DO CHILDREN DEVELOP VERTEBRAL SUBLUXATION?

Why bring your infant, child or even teenager to the Chiropractor? The easiest way to answer that question is by looking at the cause of vertebral subluxation. There are many different causes and many different responses to those causes of vertebral subluxation based on adaptation, but regardless of the specific cause or response the universal principles can be applied to infants, children and even teenagers. When looking at how vertebral subluxation can develop as early as infancy, the law of supply and demand and the law of cause and effect can also be discussed through the lens of children and stress.

As early as conception, stress can begin confronting the fetus. As discussed previously, the law of supply and demand in relation to the cause of vertebral subluxation can be applied to determine how the demand of stress alters the supply of physiological healing and whether there is adaptation or compensation to it. The law of cause and effect in relation to the cause of vertebral subluxation can be applied to determine what specific causes of stress alters the physiological response of adaptation or compensation to it. These two universal principles can be applied to the fetus through delivery and into the stages of infants, children and teenagers.

When looking at the question as to why bring your infant into the Chiropractor for a spinal analysis at such a young age, the answer to that question is because of stress and their ability to adapt to it. If they're not sufficiently adapting to their environment "stress" then they can potentially be living with vertebral subluxation within their tiny spines. The next conversation that takes place when discussing why infants and Chiropractic benefit each other is the known fact that stress confronts all ages and stages of development. Yes, even infants and babies encounter stress. Infants confront more stress than any parent gives recognition too probably because the parents are under more stress than they've ever been confronted with. Think about that concept. Most parents are trying to adapt to less sleep, more unknowns and just the physical day to day demands of having a tiny living breathing infant under their guard. With all that stress on the parents' plate, do you think the infant is experiencing any of their emotional rollercoaster and suffering from that extra stress in the household? Let's consider how stress might be negatively influencing infants right before the parent's eyes.

Have you ever been so hungry for food that your blood sugar levels drop drastically and before long your attitude and behavior turn for the worst? Our internal body chemistry has a profound impact on physiology and when babies get hungry this can become an emotional and physiological stressor on their overall well-being.

What about sleep, how is your well-being after a poor night's sleep? Sleep is vital for infants too and can become a stressor on them. To play fair, some families and infants may be adapting to this stress and growing up and developing in a great environment. Children have an amazing ability to adapt to stress, but being aware of the concept of stress and the potential threat it can play havoc on well-being over time is of key importance. For the purposes of awareness and education, there is most likely a fair percentage of infants and children compensating to the day to day demands of development and if any compensation takes place throughout the 86,000 seconds of the day-then there is a potential for vertebral subluxation to develop.

In regards to vertebral subluxation developing at an early age, the effects on their well-being may go unnoticed due to the fact that we are unable to measure the relative aspects of health and well-being. A loss of relative aspects of health and well-being at an early age may take months or years to show up as physical signs that compensation has taken place to stress. The inability to measure the loss of the relative aspects to well-being can create a false definition of well-being in our children. Our perception that if our infants and children are not suffering from physical signs of compensation to stress must indicate that they are well is not true in whole. We know with certainty that you cannot determine the quality of well-being by the degree of the presence, or absence of symptoms. If vertebral subluxation has developed as early as infancy, finding a Chiropractor with a practice that is focused on evaluating infant spines is the first step in facilitating the correction with a gentle and specific Adjustment. Why is it important for children to be evaluated by a chiropractor? This Chinese Proverb can in short answer that question when reflecting on their well-being: "The best time to plant a tree is twenty years ago, the second best time is now."

THE ADJUSTMENT ADVANTAGE FOR CHILDREN IS A PROACTIVE CHOICE TO UNLOCK THE POTENTIAL WITHIN THEIR BODY TO FUNCTION AT A HIGHER QUALITY STATE.

If you had to choose between investing into your well-being bit by bit, over time, for many years; or, not taking care of yourself for many years, leading to spending more time and money in a short amount of time to make up for lost investment opportunity, which option would you choose? If you were given a choice to invest a penny that doubles every day for 30 days, or receive one million dollars, which opportunity would provide the greater return? To break this down, on Day 1 you have $.01 and it doubles to $.02 by Day 2. Spend the next week doubling and it's valued at $.64 by Day 7. Over the next two weeks you're only at $81.92 by the end of Day 14. Once you reach Day 21, you have $10,485.76. By Day 30, you have $5,368,709.12! In this example, if you choose to double down on your consistent investments rather than instant return, you have the opportunity to receive 5 times the value! It can be easy to get caught up in the trap of instant gratification, but it is worth it to consider investing small amounts consistently over time as you can receive a greater return. How do you take care of your well-being? Do you wait until signs or symptoms are present before you choose to invest in your quality of life?

Do you consistently double down on the small decisions that can lead to exponential growth in potential benefits? How do you take care of your child's well-being? Do you wait until they have signs or symptoms present before you choose to invest into their quality of life? Do you consistently double down on small decisions that could lead to exponential growth in potential benefits for their quality of life?

3

THE ART

"The beauty about Chiropractic is the fact that it works with natural means. It puts nothing new into the body, nor does it take away any natural gland or organ. Chiropractic simply releases life forces within the body, sets free rivulets of energy over nerves, and lets nature do her work in a normal manner."

- B.J. Palmer

| 6 |

CHIROPRACTIC ADJUSTMENTS

"Adjustment means to bring into right relationship. This is what is being done in Chiropractic: bringing vertebrae into right relationship."

— Joe Strauss

HOW ARE ADJUSTMENTS FACILITATED

In order to fully grasp how The Adjustment Advantage can enhance your quality of life, it's vital to understand dynamics to The Chiropractic Adjustment.

Once vertebral subluxation is located, the next step is to introduce an applied and specific force into the spinal column or neurological system. This step is similar to Chiropractic Analysis, with different ways of producing the force and different ways of the person receiving the input. No two Chiropractic Adjustments are alike and if you've been to more than one chiropractor you likely have noticed this. The force that is introduced into the spinal column or neurological system is typically applied with high velocity and low amplitude pressure to the vertebrae.

THIS HIGH VELOCITY AND LOW AMPLITUDE PRESSURE PRODUCES
SAFE EFFECTS FOR APPLIED FORCES INTO THE BODY TO BE ADAPTED
CONSTRUCTIVELY FOR THE FACILITATION OF VERTEBRAL SUBLUXATION.

During the Chiropractic Adjustment, sometimes a joint cavitation is experienced which is an audible release of joint pressure. This noise is not an indication that the Chiropractic Adjustment has or hasn't occurred, it is just a by-product sometimes. The noises are normal within certain joints of the body and have been linked to a change in pressure within your joint during the Adjustments. The noise is referred to as a synovial fluid cavitation, or "cavitation" for short. Cavitation occurs when an applied pressure or force separates the surfaces of a synovial joint which creates a reduction in joint pressure. When the synovial joint has a reduced pressure within the cavity, the synovial fluid within the joint releases oxygen, nitrogen and carbon dioxide gasses. Those gasses that are dissolved within the solution are responsible for the pop, snap or crack noise as the gasses escape the synovial solution.

This process is similar to when you uncork a champagne bottle. Champagne contains dissolved carbon dioxide as a chemical to carbonate beverages. Carbon dioxide produces an internal pressure within beverages that are corked, and this internal pressure is released when the cork is opened and the carbon dioxide escapes the liquid. So, whether you're popping a champagne bottle or getting adjusted within a synovial joint, carbon dioxide has the chemical characteristics to make a pop, snap or crack as it escapes the liquid. After the force has been introduced into the vertebrae and surrounding tissue, a recoil within neuromusculoskeletal dynamics occurs. This neuromusculoskeletal recoil produces positive changes that the Chiropractor can utilize to determine that the body's no longer compensating to stress but rather adapting to the force that was just introduced.

The following changes can be observed in the post check: Segmental asymmetry can undergo a change towards symmetry. Abnormal passive segmental range of motion can undergo a change towards freedom from end-play restriction. Increased or working spinal musculature tone can undergo a change towards ease. Somatic sensation or perception of actual, or potential tissue damage through tenderness, discomfort or pain can undergo a change towards less severe tenderness, discomfort or pain.

WHAT IS THE ADJUSTMENT EFFECTIVENESS?

So how effective can Chiropractic Adjustments be towards your quality of life? Chiropractors utilize a deductive reasoning process when investigating the principles of self healing, well-being and practical approaches to removing interference to the body's inherent quality of life.

This act of reasoning that is characterized by or based on the conclusion of particular instances from a general law or principle allows us to make conclusions based on scientific principles that cannot be seen or measured empirically.

In short, we're creating an answer or conclusion to a new question based on an already accepted fact, principle or truth. Using this thought process is a means of creating an answer based on principles.

We can utilize deductive reasoning for the question at hand in regards to effectiveness with Chiropractic Adjustments. Deductive reasoning draws information out of that which is already true, which then makes more truth and fact within the new deduced perception. Deductive reasoning was used in our profession by starting with a major premise that cannot be denied and then logically concluding statements that must also be true by reasoning from the major premise. This process of deducing truth from a major premise was useful early on in our development of our profession while we were building certainty, but is just as powerful now as it was over one hundred years ago.

Claude Lessard, DC states in his 2017 *"A New Look at Chiropractic's Basic Science":*

"All scientific disciplines, Chiropractic, physics, chemistry, biology, psychology, etc., have basic and applied aspects. Basics science is more basic in the sense that without discovery of PRINCIPLES...there is nothing to apply. Applied science relies on and could not exist without basic science. For example, aviation uses two basic laws, the law of gravity and the law of aerodynamics and applies it to its objective which is flying. In the same way, Chiropractic uses two basic laws, the law of organization (Universal Intelligence) and the law of ACTIVE organization (Innate Intelligence) and applies its objective which is to locate, analyze and facilitate the correction of vertebral subluxations for the full express of the innate forces of the Innate Intelligence of the body."

Are Chiropractic Adjustments effective? It depends what basic principles you are utilizing as your foundation for reasoning for that question to, but if you were to utilize the definition of Chiropractic and the 33 Principles that R.W. Stephenson documented in his Chiropractic Textbook, then the answer would be YES, Chiropractic Adjustments are effective for the correction of vertebral subluxation which can create interference to the body's inherent recuperative powers and cause a state of dysfunction to well-being.

The practice of Chiropractic has a focus on the relationship between structure and function: the structure of the spine and the function of the neurological system. This structure-function relationship has an effect on your well-being that creates A Position Statement for The Adjustment Advantage.

A position statement is a viewpoint or thesis to describe one side of an arguable viewpoint, in other words, what you stand for. The position of Chiropractic is that "there is an inherent recuperative power within the body to heal itself." Your body has an innate characteristic of restoring health or strength. It naturally wants to heal damaged cells and tissues. Sometimes too much damage has occurred to the cells and tissues within the body and, therefore, healing is limited. In this case, the principle of healing and restoration is still valid, but to a lesser degree.

Chiropractors recognize limitations of healing and practice with the responsibility of working in cooperation with other health care providers for the best interest of the client. Just like limitations to healing based on the extent of the injury or trauma, so too can there be limitations to healing due to interference in the neurological system at the spinal cord level. The power to heal the body utilizes the neurological system to coordinate and direct the trillions of cells working together towards an optimal state of well-being. Your highest quality of well-being is coordinated by your neurological system through communication of mental impulses from the brain to the body and the body back to the brain through the nerves. This process needs to be free of any interference in order for an optimal state of communication and increased well-being to take place.

The practice of Chiropractic focuses on the spine due to the intimate relationship the bones of the spine have with the neurological system, which is the structure-function relationship that was mentioned earlier. The structure or alignment of your spine affects the function of the neurological system. The power within the body to heal back to an optimal state of well-being is coordinated through the neurological system, and the ability for the neurological system to function is affected by the structure or alignment of the spinal bones or vertebrate.

Chiropractic Adjustments are effective in correcting vertebral subluxation which in turn can influence the neurological function to express a higher state of well-being through the inherent recuperative power to self-heal and self-function. The effectiveness of correcting vertebral subluxation and the benefits to self-healing and self-function have limitations built within the current state of condition to the person benefiting from The Adjustment Advantage.

One question that gets brought up with effectiveness to the Chiropractic Adjustment is how does it feel? Is it painful?

No, Chiropractic Adjustments should not hurt and the purpose behind the Adjustment is to facilitate a small alteration or movement within the spinal joint that is not functioning properly so that the end result is better adaptation of spinal dynamics. The misbelief about

Chiropractic Adjustments hurting stems from a misconception about the purpose of the Chiropractic Adjustment. Receiving Chiropractic Adjustments should only focus on the spinal joints that have a state of dysfunction, a joint interfering with the neurodynamics (vertebral subluxation). Chiropractic Adjustments facilitate normal function, they should not disturb normal function within the spine. It's important to remember that Chiropractic Adjustments follow two pivotal principles in health care ethics; nonmaleficence and beneficence. Nonmaleficence is an ethical principle within health care that means do no harm intentionally. Chiropractors are all trained in their Doctorate of Chiropractic to do no harm intentionally.

Chiropractors have extensive knowledge and experience in anatomy and physiology along with proper protocols for delivering safe and effective Chiropractic Adjustments. Beneficence is an ethical principle within health care that means do good or contribute to their welfare. Personally speaking, I became a Chiropractor because I have an internal drive to help people. I would bet that most if not all Chiropractors share that similar internal drive that they want to do no harm. In Chiropractic, each Adjustment follows the principles of doing no harm and contributing to the good or welfare of the individual receiving care. To address the misconception about Chiropractic Adjustments hurting, let's discuss the process of the Chiropractic Adjustment.

Chiropractors locate and facilitate the correction of spinal joints that have characteristics of misalignment compared to the joint above or below, loss of segmental range of motion, and neurological interference to the surrounding nerve tissue. These dysfunctional joints are termed "vertebral subluxation." Subluxation can irritate the nerve tissue around the spine which can lead to a disruption in normal function within the neurological system.

When subluxation is left uncorrected, it can disrupt normal function within the body, including the joint itself. When subluxation is located and the Adjustment is facilitated, proper alignment, motion and protection of the delicate neurological system is accomplished. Chiropractic Adjustments allow the body's Innate Intelligence to restore proper relationship within the spinal joints due to the proper delivery of constructive forces being delivered by the Chiropractor. As Joseph Strauss, DC states in his 1991 *"Chiropractic Philosophy"*:

"The Adjustment is a universal force which the Innate Intelligence of the body changes (invests with new character) into an innate force. It uses that force to move a bone from the position in which the Innate Intelligence cannot move it to correct the vertebral subluxation and reduce the nerve interference to one in which it can and will correct the vertebral subluxation."

The goal with Chiropractic Adjustments is to facilitate a process from adjusting to a negative functional state to a positive functional state with each Adjustment. This process of moving from negative to positive is ingrained into our physiology since conception. In Chiropractic we refer to it as the Innate Intelligence of the body, but you could also refer to it as the law of active organization that is demonstrated throughout biology. The law of active organization within the universe applies to the human body as cells, tissues, organs and organ systems all show a level of order and structure. The unique aspect of living organisms is the ability to actively stay organized. In our body, there is an Innate Intelligence that is actively keeping us in a state of organization and vertebral subluxation is interfering with this principle. Since there is interference to this principle of active organization, there are built in mechanisms and reflexes that will attempt to self correct or self heal this dysfunctional state of tissue. No different than cutting your finger, your Innate Intelligence will start the process of healing that tissue as soon as it's damaged.

"In every living thing there is an Innate Intelligence guiding it on the path to health." —Terry Rondberg, DC

This path back to health and well-being can take place within the spine and the Chiropractor's ability to find exactly where the interference is and where they can facilitate the process back to health through a Chiropractic Adjustment.

When the Chiropractic Adjustment is facilitated alongside this inner intelligence of self correcting or self healing vertebral subluxation, the process being adjusted feels restorative and assistive. Chiropractic Adjustments should not hurt, but sometimes healing and restoration requires change and change can be symptomatic. Feeling sore, tired or just different may not be what you are looking for if you're currently compensating for stress right now, but similar to the old statement, "no pain-no gain" sometimes soreness and/or pain is a sign that healing is occuring.

Our body's active organization is always attempting to maintain an inner state of harmony and trying to adapt to the highest degree possible to those external or internal invasive forces that are breaking down cells and tissues. This inner perfection is striving for a friendly state of health and structure. It's striving for more cells and tissues that work together. Our body's inner recuperative power or Innate Intelligence is constantly striving for making the body to be as good as it possibly can be. Chiropractors strive for working alongside this process and when moving you from a state of disharmony to harmony, the Adjustment should and most often does feel restorative.

The final point to effectiveness with the Chiropractic Adjustment is how long do they last?

That's a great question and with it comes more clarity on how The Adjustment Advantage isn't something done to you, but rather a way of promoting a higher quality of life from the inner recuperative power within you. through co-creating. Each Adjustment and each person receiving the Adjustment will have different results with how long they last.

The Chiropractic Adjustment is something you co-create through an interdependence on the Chiropractor's ability to locate, analyze and facilitate the correction of areas within your spine that are out of relationship. Spinal bones are designed to protect the nerves through proper relationship with each other and the surrounding neurological tissue. If you've lost that relationship and spinal integrity is less than ideal for a working relationship, neurological disturbance from vertebral subluxation can interfere with the body's recuperative power - putting your well-being in a state of disharmony or dis-relationship. This dis-relationship and lower quality of life creates an outcome on how well you will respond to the Chiropractic Adjustment.

Within your body is the ability to self-heal, self-coordinate and self-function. Every second of your life, your body is in self-healing mode to get rid of the weak dying tissue and replenish with new healthy tissue, but that process requires time. Vertebral subluxation is a state of condition that requires healing and restoration for the spinal neurodynamics to be in proper relationship, this healing and restoration requires time. Depending upon how long vertebral subluxation has been present and how long you've been receiving Chiropractic Adjustments will be the contributing factors in how long the Adjustments last.

Chiropractic Adjustments promote proper relationship within the spinal neurodynamics, which allows the neurological tissues to function optimally and allows the body's inherent recuperative power to co-ordinate overall well-being and more self-healing. The purpose of the Chiropractic Adjustment is to promote more restoration of the tissue within your body that needs healing. In order to hold the Adjustment more effectively and in order to make the Adjustment last longer, being proactive with your lifestyle choices including your Chiropractic Care will enable the Adjustment to be more effective. Being proactive with your lifestyle choices will allow the principle of time to work in your favor and enable you to hold the Adjustments longer. So if physical, chemical and emotional stress can cause an environment for vertebral subluxation to occur, if you choose to act, create or control how you are adapting to those stressors, you're being more proactive in making the Adjustment last longer. As a reminder, these can be the contributory factors for creating an environment for vertebral subluxation:

1. Physical Stress.
2. Chemical Stress.

3. Emotional Stress.

How do you know if you're adapting or compensating to your stress and whether you're holding the Adjustment, or need to be adjusted by a chiropractor? The point of visiting your chiropractor is to let them decide through a proper evaluation for and analysis of vertebral subluxation. Malfunctioning spinal integrity can be asymptomatic and choosing to visit your chiropractor on a proactive basis based on stress levels will support the necessary Adjustment which can promote greater results for allowing them to last longer! Holding the Chiropractic Adjustment can be achieved with consistency and continuous care. Maybe you're wondering how or what you could do to help hold the Adjustments longer? If you look at the definition of "hold" several are fitting for the description as it relates to Chiropractic:

1. Keep or detain.
2. Remain secure, intact or in position without breaking or giving way.
3. Contain or be capable of containing

HOLDING THE ADJUSTMENT IS REMAINING INTACT OR IN POSITION WITHOUT BREAKING OR GIVING WAY TO EITHER THE ABILITY TO ADAPT TO STRESS OR CONTAIN OR CAPABLE OF CONTAINING YOUR CURRENT STATE OF CONDITION.

In other words, holding the Adjustment means that the positive changes that took place with your last Chiropractic Adjustment are still holding in that specific location of the spine. Irritability or disturbance to normal function is what your chiropractor can locate and analyze with their educated palpation. Their palpation can discern the difference between normal and dysfunctional neurodynamics. When the analysis points to the exact listing for vertebral subluxation, that will signify that the body's self correction was out of balance within the supply and demand. It was unable to self correct and a Chiropractic

Adjustment is necessary to introduce a force. After the Chiropractic Adjustment is facilitated, supply and demand at that segment of neurodynamics is balanced. Position and kinetic articulations within the spinal joint are functioning better, and the surrounding tissue communicates that to your chiropractor's educated palpation. After the Adjustment you walk out of your Chiropractic visit in a better state of condition and position. Fast forward a week or two of normal day to day stress and demands and you're back at your chiropractor's getting your spine evaluated for vertebral subluxation and your chiropractor states, "You're holding your last Adjustment well."

As a recap, holding the Adjustment means the following:

1. You do not require the same Chiropractic Adjustment on that specific segment as you did on your last visit.
2. You went from the last visit to the current visit without that same disturbance or irritability to the neurodynamics at that specific segment within the spine.
3. Your connective tissue and muscles didn't resort back to the same position they were fixated at on the last visit.

Holding the Chiropractic Adjustment is the name of the game and can be influenced with the following in mind: Consistency and Continuous Care are key as it relates to what can be done to help hold the Adjustments longer. If you walked into the orthodontist office, you wouldn't expect to just wear your braces for a short time or inconsistently and expect great results, you consistently wear them with repetitive modifications made in the tension of the braces for the desired position.So too with consistent and continuous Chiropractic Adjustments can the desired position and kinetic articulations be achieved. Regular Chiropractic Adjustments allows repetitive reinforcement on the ligaments, muscles and even structure of bones around the spinal cord and nerve roots to help reinforce normal position.

This repetition is similar to constantly wearing the braces with modifications to help create less severe vertebral subluxation and better spinal alignment, position and overall functionality.

In other words, holding the Adjustment! Regular Chiropractic Adjustments allow repetitive reinforcement on the ligaments, muscles and even structure of bones around the spinal cord and nerve roots to help reinforce proper relationships within the spinal neurodynamics.

ADJUSTMENT FREQUENCY

How often should I get adjusted is a common question that many times leaves a current practice member in doubt on how soon to return or someone who's never been adjusted not pursuing their first Adjustment until their in so much pain that they can't carry on with their normal activities of daily living without the aid of the benefits to the Adjustment.

Looking at this question with an ADIO perspective will allow us to better answer the question for a more consistent approach to regular Chiropractic Care.

How often should I receive Chiropractic Adjustments? Chiropractic Adjustments can be utilized either through reactive measures or a proactive investment into your overall well-being due to daily stress and demands that are pushing your body's inherent recuperative powers of self-healing to compensate rather than adapt.

The definition of proactive is "acting, creating, or controlling a situation that causes something to happen rather than responding to it after it has happened."

Being proactive doesn't mean reactive choices might not be of necessity, as well. Being reactive is natural and due to circumstances in life or limitations to healing, sometimes a reactive decision can be the best course of action that is needed.

WHEN IS THE BEST TIME TO RECEIVE A CHIROPRACTIC ADJUSTMENT
WHEN BEING PROACTIVE? THE BEST TIME TO RECEIVE A CHIROPRACTIC
ADJUSTMENT IS WHEN STRESS OUTWEIGHS THE BODY'S INNATE ABILITY
TO ADAPT TO IT.

When stress outweighs our body's innate ability to adapt, it creates an environment for vertebral subluxation to develop. How do you know if you're either adapting or compensating for the daily stressors in life? One way to know whether you're adapting or compensating is to become more cautious of stress. Being cautious means you use good judgment and are careful in practical ways. Being cautious doesn't mean you shouldn't live a life. It means you're more aware of the principle of cause and effect as it relates to your quality of life.

Appreciating the fact that stress creates an effect to our well-being and being aware of how much stress is contributing to the need for your next Chiropractic Adjustments is vital. The unique benefit to regular Chiropractic Adjustments is realizing that better adaptation to stress can occur when you're more cautious to your current stress levels and being proactive with the decision on when to next visit your chiropractor.

Here's a myth about The Adjustment Advantage: once you start going to a chiropractor, you have to keep going forever. Maybe you've heard, once you start Chiropractic, you can never stop. Another may be, you get addicted to Chiropractic. The reality? No, you do not have to keep going to the chiropractor once you start. It's your body, and ultimately, you are responsible for making the decisions that lead you towards or away from more well-being. Chiropractic can enhance your quality of life and choosing to utilize it on a regular basis can impact your choice on how far you want to take your journey towards more well-being. The misbelief about having to continue Chiropractic Care after starting can stem from a misconception about the purpose of going to a chiropractor. Before we discuss the fallacy about regular Chiropractic Care, it's important to remember that Chiropractic is within the healthcare system. One of the principles of health care ethics is autonomy, which is considered to be a fundamental practice of any health care approach. Autonomy can be defined as the ability of a person to make his or her own decisions. In Chiropractic, that means you as the consumer of the Chiropractic services must be involved in the conversation about receiving as well as returning for Chiropractic Care.

To address the misconception about having to continue on with Chiropractic Care for the rest of your life once you start, consider the viewpoint that Chiropractic can be in the same arena as healthy lifestyle choices like nutrition and exercise. If you replace nutrition or exercise with questions or concerns about continuing on after you start, you will notice a trend that points towards where the Chiropractic misconception stems from. For example, once you start eating healthy, you must eat healthy for the rest of your life. Once you start exercising, you must exercise for the rest of your life. Let's imagine that your personal trainer recommended you come back to the gym three times a week, as well as ditch fast food and replace it with good nutrition to help you reach your health goals. They would likely encourage you to incorporate these recommendations as long term lifestyle choices, and you would likely accept these recommendations.

"We are what we repeatedly do. Excellence, then, is not an act, but a habit."
—*Will Durant*

With time and repetition, the Chiropractic Adjustments can get easier and fewer due to the habit of Chiropractic Care you've created which can influence your spinal joints and neurological system to be in an optimal state. If you want to see your time and efforts pay off, create a routine for Chiropractic Care.

| 7 |

CO-CREATE A HIGHER QUALITY LIFE NOW

"Momentum is the possession of motion; requiring
effort and time to stop it. Chiropractically, Momentum is
the progress of dis-ease or health, requiring time and effort
to stop it."

— RW Stephenson

SELF REFLECT

Are you satisfied with your overall level of well-being? Are you ready to try a different approach to change your quality of life? Reinvigorate your well-being through The Adjustment Advantage by including regular Chiropractic Adjustments into your well-being routine to enhance your inner potential! What is well-being? Well-being is when you're thriving in a complete physical, mental and social state.

They say health is the greatest wealth, and your level of well-being is directly impacted by how your body is functioning. In order to thrive in a complete state, your physiological state must be functioning at its maximum capacity. What increases your well-being? We all have potential for a higher quality of life within us, but if our body is not functioning well, we do not reach that potential.

The Adjustment Advantage can enhance your inner potential by allowing your body to work closer to its maximum capacity. Chiropractic Adjustments connect you to a higher quality of physiological function by limiting interference on your neurological system caused by vertebral subluxation. Regular Chiropractic Care can also be referred to as wellness care. "Wellness" means the state of being is in good health, and may be an actively pursued goal. Our goal for you to be in a good state of health and well-being can be accomplished through recommending regular Chiropractic visits to help actively pursue a higher quality of function. Your goal for choosing regular Chiropractic Care can align with ours through the idea that how you function impacts the choices and behaviors that can support a higher quality of life. We all have choices, some choices are easier than others. Our choices lead us towards lower or higher health risks, depending on whether we choose positive or negative habits, or behaviors.

Negative behavior choices may lead to higher health risks and a lower quality of life. Positive behavior choices may lead to lower health risks and a higher quality of life. When positive behavior choices are repeated over and over it can become the key to sustaining the habit which can lead to better results. Our goal for you to be in a good state of well-being can be accomplished through making a positive behavior choice to include regular Chiropractic Care in your wellness routine. Wellness routines may attract more positive choices such as eating healthy foods, exercising more often and choosing less toxic stressors like drinking or smoking.

INCLUDING ONE POSITIVE BEHAVIOR CHOICE CAN LEAD TO MORE.

Choose regular Chiropractic Care as one way to actively pursue a higher quality of life! In order to get to where you want to be, you simply need to take the first step towards your goal. What are your well-being goals? Your goals may include exercising more, losing weight, eating healthier, or simply taking a more proactive approach to your health! A proactive approach to your well-being is about making choices that will increase your quality of life from the inside out. Regular Chiropractic Care can be one of your steps in investing in yourself from the inside out and your journey toward optimal well-being when you choose to do it consistently. Constant stress can become invasive to the body's natural ability to adapt and function. When stress wins, dysfunction can occur within the spine which chiropractors term vertebral subluxation. A specific and gentle Chiropractic Adjustment can help restore the state of dysfunction to a state of proper function.

"The future depends on what you do today." —Mahatma Gandhi

What are you doing today? Do you have plans today to do something for yourself that your future self will thank you for? They can be as simple as eating an apple or going for a walk or run. Anything today that will benefit you tomorrow is a proactive approach to your well-being. There's a balance between living in the present moment, future moment and past moments. You don't want to spend time living in the past, thinking or regretting what you did or didn't do. The balance between living in today's moment and the future moment is where the dance of proactive choices for a better future takes place. Find time throughout your day to think about who you want to become, or what you want to be doing in the future. Think about who's with you in the future, your kids, grandkids and spouse. All of these thoughts of the future should inspire you. Feelings of making wiser and better decisions today, right now for a better future tomorrow.

Where are you right now in your journey towards your optimal quality of life that you just dreamt of? If you're like most people, you have some areas where your quality of life is exceptional, some areas that are average and some areas that need immediate attention. Being aware of your current quality of life and knowing who you want to be in the future is the first step towards a future you will thank yourself for.

Now comes the step that is easiest: just do it. Just do what you need to do. Do it, do it and do it over and over again until you turn your areas of average quality choices and habits into exceptional quality decisions. Ask a professional to help you with those areas that need immediate attention and listen to their recommendations on how to benefit the most. Keep the routine and positive choices you're making right now for those areas that are going well in your life.

The next step towards your exceptional quality of life is probably the hardest step-consistently doing it day after day, week after week, month after month and year after year. This regular approach of doing the little things that matter will make your quality of life compound over time similar to an investment approach. The sooner you start the better, and the longer you do it the more rewards or gains await for you. Here's your three steps towards your future you thank you:

1. Take a self inventory of your quality of life and ask yourself what areas are great, good and bad.
2. Take action towards maintaining the great areas, improving the good areas and getting help for the bad areas.
3. Consistently practice the positive choices and habits that will promote a higher quality life over and over again to see the potential benefits that await you!

Habits and goals are much easier to stick to or achieve when we have an accountability partner. What does being an accountability partner entail? Accountability can be defined as the fact or condition of being accountable with responsibility. Being accountable is justifying your actions or decisions with someone. Are you ready to explain to someone why you are choosing actions to lead you towards a higher quality of life? There are two motives to make an Adjustment in the choices you make towards raising your quality of life:

1. Avoid pain
2. Gain pleasure.

You're either running away from something painful or running towards something positive. Due to the known fact that your health and well-being is more than how you feel, we recommend that you consider motive number 2 for the choices you make towards raising your quality of life. Choosing to gain more well-being is like eating an apple a day. It's one small piece of the puzzle that makes an impact over time. If you want to see your time and efforts pay off, create a routine for Chiropractic Care. Get started with The Adjustment Advantage and experience what a higher quality of life can produce for you!

MOMENTUM

Momentum as it relates to quality of life depends upon the philosophical state of survival values as it relates to your state of function over a given amount of time. Another way of saying it would be, gains are when your body is adapting to stress over a given period of time, and losses are when you are lacking adaptation to stress over a given period of time.Losses or a failure to adapt to stress subtracted from the gains or ability to adapt would equate your survival value in a given time period. How you're adapting to stress over a period of time is going to determine if your momentum is in favor of dis-ease or health/well-being. There is no process that does not require time and there is no time where survival to stress is necessary. No matter what you choose to do to raise your quality of life, time will always be a factor and how your adapting to stress in that time determines your momentum.

Time is always a factor and if you want to see results from what you're putting your time and energy into, try to focus on the current action that you're taking rather than the results from momentum that always takes longer than expected. Focusing on the results may shift your focus to how long it's taking to get what you want, rather than positive survival values you're building in favor of adaptational success. The results you're looking for will come with time, but it may take longer than you expected which can cause frustration and fatigue if that's where you decide to keep your focus. Consistency is key with momentum. Consistent action will move momentum in the direction of achieving your goals and getting to where you want to be over time. By focusing on the work, effort and consistent action that you're taking, it gives you confidence that positive change is taking place and momentum is in your favor.

> TIME IS ALWAYS GOING TO BE A PART OF THE PROCESS, SO REMEMBER TO ENJOY THE PROCESS TO REACH YOUR DESIRED QUALITY OF LIFE.

For those who are ready for a change in your quality of life, try to not point the finger, but instead, take responsibility for the actions that have or have not been taken. Being responsible for our own well-being is no easy task. We are constantly faced with choices that will either build up our well-being or tear it down. One way to harness momentum in your favor towards a higher quality of life is if you start looking at stress as an opportunity to become stronger by adapting to it. Look at the struggle and challenges you're facing as an opportunity to take personal responsibility for overcoming the stress in your life, and creating a stronger survival value within your physiology. The secret to stress is that the more you can adapt to the invasive forces that stress poses on your physiology, the higher your gains, or survival value can become.

No different than going to the gym everyday and increasing the amount of weights or "stress" you are bench pressing. The more weight you add to the dumbbells, the greater the resistance forces to that weight you will achieve. This process of adding muscle tissue in response to weightlifting is adaptation in the form of survival values. When utilizing this perspective towards stress, the negative challenges become a builder of momentum. Resistance builds strength and you can decide right now that your current stressors are there to build you into a stronger person because within each of us is a source of recuperative powers to adapt and heal to a higher quality of life. Look at obstacles or challenges that you're confronted with as an opportunity to take the stress and turn it into positive survival value. Situational stressors can be your barbells for a higher quality of life.

Over time, winning the warlike battle of stress vs. well-being can turn your survival values into thriving values. Your gains add up in your favor to outmatch the day to day stress that would typically beat an average gain. Your gains become too much for the stress to take on. This is no longer surviving, it's thriving. Thriving is a state of momentum over longer periods of time.

With thriving as the outcome we are all looking for, it bears witness to mention that there are times when momentum has and does go against you and your quality of life over years of lost opportunity or just pure genetic make up or chance. When challenges over time favor you or your family, this requires extra empathy for how precious our physiological states are and how our body interacts with the environment we live in.

We live in a world where we will choose today over tomorrow day after day with little thought that tomorrow may bring a new today that we cannot adapt to based on our decisions from yesterday. Living for today is normal, I do it. My family practices it. The concept that we need to make a choice that can supply us with the proper needs of today is a requirement of living in the present moment. The issue can be when we live too much in the now and not enough for the future. This creates an inability to create momentum.

Have you ever thought about what you want your quality of life to look like in the future? Do you want to be running marathons at the age of 65? Do you plan on picking up your grandchildren and rough-housing with them till they're too tired to play?

These questions are worthwhile to think about because with disregard for your future quality of life, you may be living in the quick fix reality vs. long term solution population. Our well-being is a process, not an event. This process requires momentum to work in favor of your desired state of condition.

Think about it, with major traumas being the only exception, name the last time one event caused a major shift in your quality of life. Most often it's the day by day processes that lead up to or take away from our survival values that cause a tipping point in our ability to adapt to stress and we finally hear our body asking for help for the lack of awareness to what the daily choices or lack of choices has affected to our well-being.

The processes of the day by day quick fixes can either hurt us or help us. Are you choosing an apple a day or a fast food daily? I drive by a fast food restaurant to get to work and sometimes the line for breakfast is two cars wide and 12 cars deep through the drive thru. I'm not disowning the drive thru opportunity, they are a blessing when you need them.

I'm asking you if you're asking yourself if this choice you're currently making is going to create positive or negative momentum for your well-being, and overall function in the future. Not today, but for the future. What will this choice do for your well-being tomorrow?

Start looking at your well-being as a bundle of little choices that you make to either add or take away your survival values. Not only are our choices adding to or taking away, but so too is the daily stress affecting the performance of well-being.

The consistent choices we make each day and the consistent stress our body needs to adapt to slowly moves the pendulum of balance and harmony to your inner well-being.

To take it back to physics class, a pendulum works by converting energy back and forth, similar to a rollercoaster ride. When the bob is highest or furthest from the ground, it has maximum stored energy or what science calls potential energy. When the bob swings or oscillates back and forth, it consistently switches its energy back and forth between potential and kinetic.

Potential energy is the stored energy within an object or you because of its position. Kinetic energy is related to the object or your ability to move and in its immediate environment and can be transferred from one moving object to another.

Why all the physics conversation? Think about your quality of life or well-being within your body as a pendulum or the bob that is moving to the left and right, up and down. When the bob is at its lowest point that represents when your body is dysfunctional and has a lack of wholeness and when the bob is to the left or to the right at its highest point that represents wholeness, function and well-being.

We go back and forth every day and the body's innate intelligence is striving to keep the balance between the lows and the highs. Striving for momentum towards the highest state of potential energy. Since well-being is largely regulated by your neurological system and your neurological system plays a vital role in adapting to stress, how your nerves function play a factor to how your pendulum swings.

Chiropractors are concerned about the performance of your neurological system because the vertebrae that surround and protect the nerves can become displaced and interfere with the mental impulses that travel through the nerves and supply your body with the ability to adapt and survive based on the consistent choices you're making for today or tomorrow.

The Adjustment Advantage can move your body towards wholeness and well-being allowing that pendulum to swing away from the lows and closer to the inner potential energy that's waiting to be expressed. This is adaptation. Where your focus goes, energy flows! Or in other words, where your momentum goes, your energy flows.

Life is energy, and energy is never stagnant — it's in constant flux and movement. The energy source to your well-being is how chiropractic can promote whole body benefits. Focusing on the principle that your body generates and coordinates well-being through energy is a step in the direction of living life at a higher quality.

With the brain being the source of your life energy, it sends energy down the spinal cord and then out to your entire body through the nerves. This cycle then repeats back from the body through the nerves up the spinal cord and into the brain. This cyclical flow of energy from brain to body and body back to brain through your neurological system is how your trillions of cells work together physiologically.

When any of the 24 vertebrae subluxate out of proper position and irritate rather than protect the nerves, interference in the transmission of neurological life sustaining energy, or impulses can occur between your brain and body.

THE CORRECTION OF VERTEBRAL SUBLUXATION IS ACCOMPLISHED THROUGH THE ADJUSTMENT ADVANTAGE, SIMILAR TO TURNING THE DIMMER UP ON THE LIGHT SWITCH ALLOWING MORE LIGHT TO SHINE.

The Adjustment Advantage assists the vertebrae into normal alignment with gentle pressure in a specific line of drive. Chiropractic Adjustments open up the circuit between the brain and body by creating less interference in the neurological system, allowing normal function to occur throughout the entire body due to adequate nerve supply. Being free from vertebral subluxation will benefit your quality of life to the degree it's affected by your neurological system. Chiropractors advocate more well-being or a higher quality life through the application of Chiropractic Adjustments, which remove interference in the life energy traveling through your nerves.

We all have two approaches when it comes to utilizing Chiropractic Adjustments. The first approach is utilizing the positive influence Chiropractic Adjustments has on well-being so your self-healing characteristics can overcome a specific health condition or symptoms. This approach does not necessarily mean your Chiropractor is specifically treating your health condition. It also does not mean your Chiropractor is trying to reduce your symptoms. In general, this approach is common within Chiropractic because when the focus is on correcting vertebral subluxation, the positive influence on your whole well-being can be attained and health conditions and symptoms often are replaced with function and well-being.

You may have no signs or warnings that your well-being is dysfunctional. Your overall state of condition may feel fine, but only using Chiropractic Care to get you to this point of feeling fine is similar to saying "Pick the low-hanging fruit first." In regards to health and well-being, going for the easiest way to feeling better or a quick fix can be just that. It's quick and the amount of labor you put into it is what you'll get in return. Apple picking is practiced from the top to the bottom in order to allow the heavily shaded fruit to ripen and allow the low-hanging fruit more time to ripen.

Using Chiropractic Adjustments to feel better is similar to picking the low-hanging fruit first; it may suffice for one or two apples, but it won't produce a sack of ripened apples that will allow you to eat an apple a day.

The second approach and the position of The Adjustment Advantage is focusing on utilizing the positive influence Chiropractic Adjustments has on well-being so your self-healing characteristics can adapt to stress with promotion for an optimal state of well-being through the expression of the body's Innate Intelligence. This approach is a consistent approach or lifestyle of maintaining a higher state of well-being.

This approach is what I refer to as Regular Chiropractic Care. Regular Chiropractic Care is a proactive approach to evaluating the state of condition of your spine regardless of the presence or absence of symptoms. Oftentimes, symptoms just don't correlate to how well your physiology is functioning. Regular Chiropractic Care is about consistency and consistency is a key to success in creating positive momentum.

When utilizing Regular Chiropractic Care, your focus tends to go towards the potential benefits that await for you as the reward rather than focusing on the low hanging fruit for today's apple. Focusing in on consistent Chiropractic Adjustments with respect to the ups and downs to how the body is expressing states of adaptation allows the inner recuperative power of the body to consistently generate more momentum towards a higher state of well-being. Consistent states of more well-being allows for greater ways to adapt to stress which in turn allows your well-being to not be drained or lost due to the demands of the day to day stress.

As a practicing Chiropractor for over ten years, my practice is primarily full of the second category of consumers of Regular Chiropractic Care. My clients visit our practice on a weekly basis with the focus on more well-being and greater adaptability to the day to day stress. In general, our results in life are dependent upon where our focus is and our quality of life is no different.

If your quality of life is not where you want it to be, try monitoring where your focus is. Reflect on what you focus on and why you are focusing on it. Associate more positive results or less negative consequences with a specific behavior.

When you take control of your focus, you take control of your life! Associating positive rewards and negative consequences to your focus can push and pull you in the direction of where you want your quality of life to be.

The key to a higher quality life is making choices and decisions during the day that will not only benefit today, but also provide a long term solution to keep that pendulum in positive momentum. Short term choices for today may be necessary at times, but the future needs to be kept in mind so the pendulum doesn't become out of balance with little to no momentum in your favor.

Quick fixes to make you feel better today may move that pendulum back into motion, but soon enough or over time if the choices and the stress are slowing the speed of motion down your pendulum can end back up in the low slow speed of transfer or out of balance.

Consider consistency and positive choices for what the future you will benefit from as a long term solution for keeping your pendulum in motion towards the potential for more well-being or higher quality life. These consistent choices align with The Adjustment Advantage.

Regardless of what your current state of well-being is right now, you have two approaches toward its state tomorrow: momentum towards positive adaptation to life's stressors or towards compensation and disharmony. Life constantly throws difficulties and challenges towards us, choose to find ways to adapt to life's stressors. Choose to take personal responsibility for your current state of momentum. Every decision you've made up to this point in your current state has brought you to where you are now. Look forward and find ways today to become stronger so big momentum can swing in your favor.

COMMIT-COOPERATE-CONSISTENCY

Here are 3 ways to help make The Adjustment Advantage work for you:

1. Commit to making your future better than the past.
2. Cooperate with your chiropractor's professional recommendations for care.
3. Consistently and deliberately take action steps to include Chiropractic into your routine.

Do you have your Chiropractic visit in your agenda? If not, why don't you? Do you find that you are too busy? Being too busy is an even greater reason to have an agenda that helps set the tone for your day/week. Find time at the start of your week to prioritize the major goals that need to be accomplished. Once you have a list of what needs to be done, the next step is finding a day and time to include those priorities in your schedule. Choosing to include Regular Chiropractic Care in your agenda can be a positive habit towards a higher quality of life. Positive habits are a necessity in today's demanding world, but we don't always do what's positive for ourselves. What's easy to do is also easy not to do. We know that eating good food, getting adequate rest and exercising are positive habits that raise your well-being. But how many of us skip a day or week in these positive habits?

Consistency and adding our positive habits to our agenda is key in our success. Practice these habits at the same time of day, each day, or same day of the week, each week. In regards to Chiropractic, choose a day of the week that works for you to visit your chiropractor, let's say that day is Tuesdays. Each Tuesday, find a time in the day when you are able to block off time for yourself. Now hit repeat on your appointment, and practice this for 60 days. It takes 60 days of consistently doing the same positive habit to make it stick. Regular Chiropractic Care can be a part of your secret to raising your well-being if you turn it into a habit. Today's stressful, demanding way of living will try to take you out of your routine and into a state of chaos. Stick to your agenda and don't lose sight of the habits that create the most positive impact on your well-being. Regular Chiropractic Care can be a worthwhile investment of time in your agenda! In order to achieve optimal results from regular Chiropractic Care we recommend commitment, cooperation and consistency. Commit to making your future better than the past. Cooperate with your chiropractors' professional recommendations for care.

TAKE CONSISTENT AND DELIBERATE ACTION STEPS TOWARDS INCLUDING REGULAR CHIROPRACTIC CARE INTO YOUR LIFESTYLE.

If you hold yourself accountable to these three C's on a regular basis, you will see the benefits from Chiropractic Care that will make the reward outweigh the investment. Can you make the commitment to regular Chiropractic Care right now?

Chiropractic Care is a great approach to invest into your overall well-being through this inside-out viewpoint of health. Hindsight is 20/20. In other words, it's easier to look back with "20/20 vision" and evaluate the decisions you made, than to predict the outcomes that will take place in the future. Benefiting from The Adjustment Advantage can be similar. It's easier to look back on consistent care and see the value of each Chiropractic Adjustment than it is to predict what good will come from future visits to your chiropractor. Chiropractic Hindsight is when you've been under regular Chiropractic Care and can see the value in each Adjustment that has produced higher quality life for you. For those who use Chiropractic consistently, there may likely be obvious indicators before and after the Adjustment that demonstrate that it's a worthwhile investment.

What about those who have never been to a chiropractor before? What if they're interested in learning more about it, or even considering trying it? How do you encourage someone to do something without forecasting what the future holds for them while they're under care?

Steve Jobs has a famous quote, "You can't connect the dots looking forward; you can only connect them looking backwards. So you have to trust that the dots will somehow connect in your future. You have to trust in something — your gut, destiny, life, karma, whatever."

In Chiropractic, we like to trust that the "Adjustments will connect" in your future through a logical conclusion that each Chiropractic Adjustment can provide a positive influence to your well-being and quality of life. This logic is derived from the evidence that spinal health is linked to the condition of the brain and neurological system. Poor spinal health affects your neurological well-being. Over 120 years of Chiropractic hindsight continues to produce connections between the relationship of structure and function. When there is proper spinal structure, neurological function is impacted and the innate recuperate powers to heal and coordinate proper function are fully expressed. So, how do you know if you need to be adjusted by a chiropractor? Always consult with a chiropractor who will help determine that care is appropriate for you. This process includes a consultation, as well as a biomechanical and neurophysiological evaluation to make a determination of the need for care. Based on findings in the evaluation, this process may be followed by the Chiropractic Adjustment.

Everyday, our body naturally heals and repairs itself for the overall ability to stay in a state of well-being. The process of healing and regeneration of new cells and tissues is an amazing process and needs very little assistance to function in a state of well-being. However, all good things have limitations. Due to limitations of matter, our body can only repair and create new healthy cells and tissues at a rate that is reflected by the choices you make for your well-being. Choices like doing something positive for yourself, doing something negative for yourself or doing nothing. Negative choices in this case can also be referred to as stress. If too much stress is put on your body, there can inevitably be a breaking point to the process of healing and restoration. Positive choices allow for adaptation to the negative stress that we encounter. By making positive choices for your body when you are faced with stress and high demands, you can help increase your overall well-being and stay ahead in health.

Due to our highly demanding lifestyles that are full of stress and chaos, positive choices are recommended that promote more well-being for your body and assist in adaptation to get ahead of stress. Choosing The Adjustment Advantage for a higher quality of life is a proactive choice that can help your body stay ahead of demands and stress. When making the choice to get your spine evaluated for vertebral subluxation, you're making a proactive choice to improve your state of well-being.

The Adjustment Advantage is a great way to enhance vitality, no matter your age! Millions of people utilize Chiropractic each year to raise their quality of life. Now take what you learned and choose Regular Chiropractic Care! The hardest part about a routine is getting started. Here are 3 steps you can take to be the catalyst of your Chiropractic routine:

1. Identify Your Day(s) of the Week to Visit Your Chiropractor. We find that clients who create a consistent schedule of visiting us on the same day(s) of the week tend to be more consistent with their visits due to the habit that has been created. When you make a habit and stick to it, you can hold yourself accountable to checking it off your priority list. For example, if you have a habit of exercising three times a week and you miss a day in your weekly routine, you'll feel inclined to make up that visit, or know that you didn't accomplish your goals for that week which will push you to get in your three visits the following week.

2. Identify Your Goal(s) from Chiropractic Care. Create an inspiring goal to push you through the ups and downs of creating your Chiropractic routine. Life will, likely, take you out of your routine and the good habits you're trying to create. Find a motivation that will pull you back on track towards success. If you need to pick up your kids from school on the day you typically visit your chiropractor one week, and the following week you go on vacation, you now have two weeks worth of motivating rea-

sons to pull you back into the rhythm of consistent Chiropractic Care. One goal that clients may have when they start care is the ability to perform better in their day to day functions at work, like computer work for longer periods of time. When you realize that investing into your well-being is an investment into your job performance, your goal to thrive during the day, rather than merely survive, will power you back into your regular routine.

3. Identify the Impact from Your Chiropractic Routine on Those Around You Taking care of yourself to take care of your priorities can benefit not only yourself, but also those around you. When you are functioning better, you can serve those in your inner circle who you have close relationships with. Think of those closest to you to help inspire you towards the consistent habit of regular Chiropractic Care. Chiropractic Care can help restore a proper relationship within the spinal joints which can enhance the innate recuperative power of the body to function in its normal state. When dysfunction is located within the spine due to vertebral subluxation, the communication can be less than optimal between brain and body, in turn, creating a lower quality of function. The integrity of your spinal joints can enhance the innate recuperative power of the body to heal itself due to the emphasis on the relationship between structure and function that is coordinated by the neurological system.

ACKNOWLEDGMENTS

I'd like to open these Acknowledgements with a quote by one of my dear mentors, "If you are not out to change the world, everything else is Mickey Mouse." -Reggie Gold

This book would not have been created if it wasn't for Reggie Gold's efforts to teach students and Chiropractors that Chiropractic doesn't need a Philosophy, Chiropractic is a Philosophy-thank you Reggie.

Joseph Strauss, this book could not have been completed if I didn't have the inspiration and the goal to continue to carry on the torch you lit with your Blue Book Publications. I appreciate your mentorship and contribution to the profession. Thank you for being a friend and mentor in time of need, I am grateful for you!

Looking back on the amount of time it took me to compile my thoughts into this publication, each hour writing was spent working towards building our brand message at ChiroWay Chiropractic. If it weren't for our founding ChiroWay Franchisee's this book would have taken several more years to compile. Thank you: Michael Madison, DC Drew Fautsch, DC Lance Baumgard, DC Danielle Berger, DC Tom Stecker, DC Blake Bredeson, DC Austin Murdock, DC Nick Lundbohm, DC

As I was drafting this book, each and every member of ChiroWay, especially ChiroWay of Woodbury, deserves to be acknowledged as you served as the purpose to educating you and shining the light on Chiropractic and all the beautiful benefits it has waiting for your to attain as you visit us week in and week out year after year. Thank you!

With a full time practice and a franchise to run, completing a project like this couldn't be accomplished without the team members who contribute to the companies like it's their own. At the forefront of those team members is Natalie Lewis. Thank you for finishing all of my projects I started, including this publication. You are the hardest worker I know and your grind on the editing, layout, design and future marketing of this book deserve special acknowledgement. Thank you! I look forward to getting started on the second book with your contribution! Special shout out to our newest team members that have taken the lead on serving our members at ChiroWay of Woodbury to allow me to devote the necessary time to projects like this, thank you Angela Ross and Matt Hill, DC for joining our family at ChiroWay. We appreciate your contribution to this book by keeping our members well adjusted so they can experience The Adjustment Advantage. Also, Angela you have a gift with your camera, thank you for adding your artistic contribution to the front cover! Libby Varnum, thank you for your behind the scenes help with this publication!

Finally, I would like to conclude this Acknowledgement with a special recognition to whom I work tirelessly for. They have my truest appreciation for giving me an opportunity to work day and night on the craft that I love and cherish. Thank you for supporting my passion for Chiropractic. Laura, Tristan and Laila-this book would not be possible if I didn't have you to work hard for and for you to allow me to work so hard for you. Laura, thank you for allowing me to pursue my passion and believing in me and for supporting ChiroWay in its infancy years when it needed someone like to you whip it into shape! Tristan and Laila, thank you for your consistent willingness to receive The Adjustment Advantage from your dad. This publication is an extension of my efforts to see more people benefit from Regular Chiropractic Care so they too can experience The Adjustment Advantage like you do. Watching my children grow up with Regular Chiropractic Care has been one of the greatest sources of clarity and conviction to the potential benefits within The Adjustment Advantage. For the rest of my immediate family members who pushed me to be me, thank you and I acknowledge how our time together has inspired me to have a family to work hard for and leave a legacy for years to come. Thank you Mom, Dad, Tyler and Tony, Tom, June and Tony. You all deserve to be in my dearest appreciation for contributing to the cause behind this first book. One more recognition for my mother, the years of motherly love and filling my bucket with positive affirmations has and will last a lifetime for me. This book is an effort of giving it back to those who need to hear positive affirmations like I did when I was younger. Thank you and I love you!

RESOURCES

Gold, Reggie. *The Triune of Life*. Sherman College of Straight Chiropractic, 1998

Lessard, Claude. *A New Look at Chiropractic's Basic Science*. Lessard Chiropractic Centre, 2017.

Stephenson, Ralph W. *The Chiropractic Textbook*. The Author, 1948.

Strauss, Joseph B. *Chiropractic Philosophy*. Foundation for the Advancement of Chiropractic Education, 1994.

Strauss, Joseph B. *Enhance Your Life Experience*. Foundation for the Advancement of Chiropractic Education, 1996.

DISCLAIMER

All content found in this publication, including: title, text, advice, or benefits were created for informational purposes only. The title is not stating any chiropractic practice, chiropractor, treatment or advice in this publication is more favorable or superior position; but rather when receiving Chiropractic Care one has an opportunity to gain a higher quality life or a favorable circumstance of lesser vertebral subluxation-the benefit. The information in this book is not intended to diagnose, mitigate or prescribe the use of any technique as a form of treatment for any physical conditions, symptoms or diseases. Directly consult with a qualified health care professional for any medical or chiropractic questions or advice. All information and resources found in this publication are based on the opinions of the author and are meant to motivate and inform readers to make their own health decisions after consulting with their health care provider. In addition to the opportunity to gain a higher quality life or benefits of Chiropractic Care, one should also be aware of the existence of some risks. Risks associated with some Chiropractic Care may include soreness, musculoskeletal sprain/strain, and fracture. In addition, there have been reported cases of stroke associated with Chiropractic Care. Research and scientific evidence does not establish a cause and effect relationship between Chiropractic Care and the occurrence of stroke; rather studies indicate that people may be consulting chiropractors when they are in the early stages of a stroke. In essence, there is a stroke already in process. However, you are being informed of this reported risk. Trying to manipulate your own spine in an attempt to facilitate a Chiropractic Adjustment on yourself is not recommended. People may have the urge to "crack" their own spine in the hopes they'll receive momentary relief from the stiffness, tension or pain that they are experiencing. If self-manipulation turns into a habit of temporary relief, problems can occur due to the potential negative effects this practice can create on the soft tissue ligaments, muscles and even facet joints. The author does not recommend or endorse any specific technique or form of treatment, Chiropractor, products, procedures, opinions, or other information that may be mentioned in this publication.

CPSIA information can be obtained
at www.ICGtesting.com
Printed in the USA
LVHW080825090921
697390LV00002B/8/J